CW01072450

Prevention is Better than Cure:
History of the Cork University Dental
School and Hospital, 1913–2013

PREVENTION IS BETTER THAN CURE

*History of the Cork University Dental
School and Hospital, 1913–2013*

John Borgonovo, Denis O'Mullane & Tim Holland

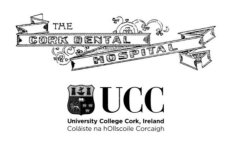

University College Cork, Ireland
Coláiste na hOllscoile Corcaigh

First published in 2013 by
Cork University Dental School and Hospital
University College Cork
Cork
Ireland

© John Borgonovo, Denis O'Mullane & Tim Holland, 2013

All rights reserved. No part of this book may be reprinted or reproduced or utilised in any electronic, mechanical or other means, now known or hereafter invented, including photocopying and recording or otherwise, without either the prior written permission of the publisher or a licence permitting restricted copying in Ireland issued by the Irish Copyright Licensing Agency Ltd, 25 Denzille Lane, Dublin 2.

The right of John Borgonovo, Denis O'Mullane & Tim Holland to be identified as authors of this work has been asserted by them in accordance with Copyright and Related Rights Acts 2000 to 2007.

ISBN 978-0-9927244-0-5

Layout: Dominic Carroll, Ardfield, Co. Cork
Printing: Brunswick Press Ltd, Dublin

CONTENTS

FOREWORD

*T*ODAY, University College Cork is a world-class research university, dedicated to excellence in teaching and learning. Sometimes, knowing where we came from can tell us where we are going. The centenary anniversary of the foundation of the Cork University Dental School and Hospital (CUDSH) offers UCC one such retrospective opportunity.

I approached Emeritus Professor Denis O'Mullane to write the history of the Cork University Dental School and Hospital on the premise that when you want to get something done, you ask a busy person. Denis is one of the most respected figures in Irish dental scholarship, and has been a devoted servant to UCC since his student days. Fortunately, he has proved himself as successful a historian as he has been a researcher and educator. For this project Denis secured two co-authors, Tim Holland and Dr John Borgonovo. Tim Holland is a retired consultant in paediatric dentistry and a long-time CUDSH teacher and administrator. Like Denis, Tim is also a CUDSH graduate. John Borgonovo is a historian in the School of History at UCC, specialising in twentieth-century Irish and Cork history. Together, they have managed to describe a century of UCC dental education in an informative and entertaining way.

The authors consistently place CUDSH in a broader context, as readers learn about evolutions in dentistry, third-level education, and Irish political and social life. Fundamentally, this book highlights the many challenges overcome at CUDSH since its foundation in 1913. Along the way, CUDSH became a crucial health-care resource for generations of residents of the city and county of Cork. It developed a research capacity that is internationally recognised by universities, governments and private industry. Throughout its history, the dental school has also produced hundreds of talented graduates who have achieved professional success in Ireland and around the globe. As this book makes clear, such achievements stemmed from an extensive and interconnected school community that continued to push CUDSH throughout the century. Theirs is a remarkable tale of motivated students, inspired staff and institutional resilience.

This book is not only about CUDSH, dental education or UCC. It is also a tale of people with passion and determination, who overcame high odds to achieve their goals. As such, it will be appreciated by readers far beyond UCC's dental family, as well as those within its embrace.

Dr Michael Murphy
President, University College Cork

ACKNOWLEDGEMENTS

THIS book was a collaborative process, and could not have happened without the full support of current and former staff and students of Cork University Dental School and Hospital. The authors would also like to acknowledge additional contributions and assistance received during this undertaking.

Thanks are due to Attracta Halpin, registrar of the National University of Ireland, for providing access to NUI governing-body material. At UCC, the Special Collections staff in the Boole Library were very helpful, especially Sheyeda Allen, Mary Lombard and Peadar Cranitch. Thanks also to University archivist Catriona Mulcahy, who frequently lent her office space and expertise to our archival work. The UCC Student Records and Examination Office staff proved very accommodating, while Nancy Hawkes of UCC Media and Marketing offered her own valued advice on the publishing process. The staff of Ionad Bairre – UCC's Teaching and Learning Centre – were accessible and helpful. We would also like to acknowledge Michael Hanna of the College of Medicine and Health for sharing his knowledge of John Woodroofe and the Cork School of Anatomy. Special appreciation should also be expressed to the entire staff of the Oral Health Services Research Centre, who frequently devoted their time, skills and facilities to the project. Professor John Higgins, head of the College of Medicine and Health at UCC, provided key assistance during a critical period. Professor Finbarr Allen fully supported this book from its inception, and acted as a trusted adviser throughout the project. We are grateful to Finbarr and Kathryn Neville for acting as readers of the final manuscript.

The Munster branch of the Irish Dental Association generously allowed access to its records, which was facilitated by Judith Phelan (BDS 1988) and Fiona Twohig (BDS 2002). Thanks also to Denise McCarthy (BDS 1977), who donated her copy of the 'save the school' petition from her own archives. We are also grateful to David O'Flynn, chief officer and registrar of the Dental Council, for his assistance.

On the production level, Dominic Carroll of Ardfield, west Cork, designed and laid out the book. He also provided superb editorial services, and acted as a trusted adviser on the publishing process. J.P. Quinn, head of UCC Visitors' Centre, offered critical assistance with the retail and sales side of publication, and has kindly made the book available for sale at the UCC gift shop. We are grateful for the generous supply of photographs provided by Ger Fitzgerald, P.J. Byrne and Neil Nash.

Finally, we would like to recognise the vital role played by Kate McSweeney of UCC, who provided administrative support and frequently acted as project manager. She kept the entire endeavour on schedule, while tracking and organising countless contributions and submissions. Kate lent her marketing expertise in the weeks and months preceding the book launch. Her organising acumen and constant good cheer made her a very welcome addition to the book-project team.

1

FOUNDATIONS

----

*T*HE Cork University Dental School and Hospital (CUDSH) was founded by a confluence of local, national and international events during the early years of the twentieth century.

Internationally, dentistry was becoming professionalised, following similar advances in modern medicine across the industrial world. Nationally, Britain and Ireland were moving towards a fully qualified dental profession. Locally, University College Cork was experiencing an ambitious growth programme under perhaps its most dynamic and influential president. Together these factors produced a dental school and hospital that has endured for one hundred years.

THE INDUSTRIAL REVOLUTION & MEDICINE

Medical historians classify the fifty years from 1880 to 1930 as the critical period in the emergence of the modern medical profession. Before this time, medical practitioners competed against numerous alternative healers. Hospitals functioned primarily as charitable welfare institutions for the poor, rather than as educational and scientific centres. The medical marketplace was essentially unregulated, and the training of medical professionals varied widely.

During the second half of the nineteenth century, the Industrial Revolution brought massive economic and social change to Europe and North America. Factory employment drew large segments of the rural population into urban areas, where intense poverty became a visible and often unhealthy issue for the middle and upper classes. The spread of illness and social problems beyond their normal social confines created a demand for improvements in public health. State-financed health treatment, medical education and public-health measures followed.

Technical innovation associated with the Industrial Revolution also improved medical technology, which made health-care treatment increasingly sophisticated. As a result, medical practitioners required more advanced and standardised training. By the last decade of the nineteenth century, governments, medical professionals and universities collaborated to create degree programmes. University medical degrees became required to practise medicine. As a result, qualified professionals further outdistanced untrained practitioners, whose ranks included quacks who often endangered patients and brought medicine into disrepute. Professionalisation improved medical practitioners' social respectability, reduced competition with alternative medicine, increased incomes, and provided a voice in public-health policy. Similarly, university qualifications became standard during this period for such professions as teaching, civil engineering, veterinarian medicine and pharmacy. Professional associations created registers of members in good standing, which the public and later the state came to regard as necessary for practice.

In medicine, credentials ensured patients received competent and ethical treatment above a minimum standard. At the same time, fear of unhealthy urban living produced an international obsession with good health and bodily discipline. Organised sports and a 'playground movement' emerged during these same decades, as did health recreation, such as spa treatments, public baths, swimming and gymnastics. In addition, mandatory schooling created mass literacy, which gave rise to modern advertising. Newspaper and magazine adverts for beauty and health-care products fed consumer demand for medical treatment. Dentistry was one of many fields of medicine to benefit from these social changes.

MODERN DENTISTRY

For centuries, dental care had been the domain of both trained dentists and untrained tooth extractors. Preventive dentistry was virtually unknown, and extraction was often left to barbers, blacksmiths or self-taught specialists. The dental profession was on a lower social standing than medicine, and worked on an apprentice-ship basis. Dental practitioners took on apprentices for a number of years, passing on basic knowledge while retaining a few trade secrets from potential competitors. However, modern society's new challenges changed the profession in the mid-nineteenth century. Dentistry quickly followed medicine by embracing professionalisa-tion and higher-education qualifications.

The Industrial Revolution also changed dental health among the public. Mass-produced factory goods transformed popular nutrition. Sugar consumption increased by up to seven hundred per cent as chocolate, biscuits, jams, cocoa and other sweet products seeped into the populace. Dental decay and infection became a more serious and visible problem in newly urbanised nations, which encouraged eventual government action. The promotion of dental products, especially toothpaste, also increased the public's desire for dental treatment.

Meanwhile, scientific discovery associated with the Industrial Revolution rapidly improved techniques and technology used in dentistry. The introduction of ether and nitrous oxide allowed for sophisticated operations, while procaine (now commonly known as Novocaine) became a local anaesthetic. Plaster of Paris was intro-duced in 1844, and used for teeth impressions. In the 1850s hand drills with steel bur heads became common, while the heating of gold foil – a property known as cohesion – improved filling materials. Zinc phosphate, introduced to dentistry in 1879, was a major advancement as a cementing agent and filling material. Louis Pasteur and Robert Koch's work in the 1860s exposed the nature of microorganisms, which led to infection-control measures such as the sterilisation of instruments. In the same decade, Joseph Lister's germ theory of disease gained acceptance, introducing the 'antiseptic era' (today, he is popularly remembered for the antiseptic mouthwash Listerine). Around the same time, Sanfard Barnum introduced the rubber dam to allow dryness required for cohesive gold restorations. In 1871 Morrison introduced the foot-treadle dental engine, a foot-operated device that increased rotational speed used in drills. A few years earlier, Morrison produced his first dental chair, which he improved in 1877 by installing pump-type hydraulics. The discovery of electricity in the late 1800s led to electric (battery-operated) drills, and eventually to modern high-speed drills. In the 1890s G.V. Black introduced scientific cavity preparation, and Wilhelm Conrad Röntgen discovered X-rays.

Technical sophistication required better training. Formal dental education had begun in the United States. The Baltimore College of Dental Surgery opened in 1839, and within a few years nearly two dozen similar schools were operating. University-affiliated dental schools and dental degree programmes began at Harvard University in 1867, and were quickly followed at major schools such as the University of Michigan and the University of Pennsylvania (the latter's most famous graduate was the Old West gunfighter, John 'Doc' Holliday). Formal dental education emerged in Canada during the same decades, as did professional dental journals. However, Europe was slower to formalise degree programmes.

The new profession of dentistry still faced public scepticism and competition from untrained tooth extractors. One notorious char-latan was the supposed Native American medicine man Sequah. According to one historian, Sequah and his entourage dressed in Native American or cowboy costumes. Sequah extracted teeth quickly, and often worked alongside a brass band to drown out any cries from uncomfortable patients. He proved so popular he created a Sequah franchise, selling the persona to imitators operat-ing in Britain and Ireland. The 1890 visit to Cork city by Sequah produced bedlam. Appearing at the Cork Cornmarket, Sequah was confronted by University College Cork medical students. Seemingly intending to simultaneously defend the medical pro-fession and engage in a student prank, they shouted down Sequah and insulted his curing agents. Ejected by the police, the rowdy

THE FIRST DENTAL X-RAY MACHINE IN CORK

One of the dental hospital's most notable early achievements was its installation of a dental X-ray machine, which the reliable Cork dental historian Ray Gamble believed was the first in Ireland. The acquisition was proposed in January 1922 by Israel Scher at a meeting of the dental-school staff held in the practice of Dean M.B. Pericho at 3 South Mall. Scher argued that an X-ray machine was essential to hospital operations and student training. Though a general X-ray machine remained available at the North Infirmary, Scher considered a custom-made dental apparatus far superior. It would also enable students to learn how to take and read X-rays on-site. To fund the purchase, Scher explained that private-practice dentists in Cork could be charged a usage fee. Scher passed out literature on his preferred machine, the Ritter Dental X-ray Unit. Intrigued, the hospital asked de Trey & Company for a cost estimate, including installation, though a final purchase decision was deferred until the next staff meeting.

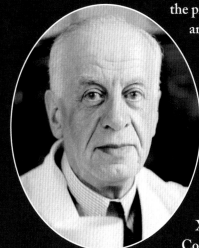

Israel 'Issa' Scher, dean of CUDSH, 1933–49.
COURTESY DR EDDIE SCHER

Two weeks later, the persistent Scher requested permission to launch a campaign to secure funding. When some members questioned the likelihood of a grant from the North Infirmary, Scher offered to canvas governing-board members and educate them about the machine. Dean Pericho supported the £400 Scher initiative, having been convinced that the apparatus would essentially pay for itself. With a charge of five shillings per sitting and used an average of four times per week, Scher estimated an annual income of nearly £50. To cover any possible shortfalls, Scher asked the staff to be prepared to pay £2 annually, which they agreed to. Scher and Michael Hunt were delegated to secure permission from the hospital governing body. One member suggested that if Scher succeeded in getting the machine installed, a medal should be 'struck up for him'.

The following month, Scher and Hunt visited de Trey's in London for a demonstration of the machine. The company also offered to underwrite a small annual prize, which became the de Trey Prize, awarded to the 'best attempt' at setting up a full upper and lower denture on an articulator.

At Hunt's suggestion, a new X-ray room was created by dividing the students' room in two. Scher had accurately predicted the machine's cost-effectiveness, as it soon provided the hospital with a small but steady profit. Less satisfactory from Scher's point of view was the filling of a new hospital radiologist position. At a meeting in May 1922, Scher nominated himself, explaining how 'he had gone into Radiology minutely' and learned how to operate the new machine. However, for unexplained reasons the staff elected Hunt to the radiologist position. Scher's feelings about the decision can be guessed at by his absence from dental-hospital staff meetings for the next six months. Three years later, Scher became the hospital's consulting radiologist, though Michael Hunt still headed the Radiology Department. Hunt held that position for thirty-seven years, until his death in 1959. The long-retired Israel Scher did not apply for the vacancy.

students then marched to the homes of their medical professors and cheered for 'science', but were dispersed by a threatened baton charge from a force of Royal Irish Constabulary. In Cork and beyond, the day of the unqualified extractor was drawing to a close.

In 1860 the Royal College of Surgeons created the Licentiate in Dental Surgery (LDS). The Dentists Act of 1878 established a register of dental practitioners, which further popularised the LDS in Britain and Ireland. Now, only licensed practitioners could use the title 'dentist' or 'dental surgeon', though unlicensed dentists could advertise themselves as 'dental consultants' or 'dental experts'. Educational programmes were required to provide the LDS qualification, with the Royal Dental Hospital acting as an examining body. The newly established British and Irish dental associations maintained professional standards and oversaw the awarding of credentials.

A DENTAL SCHOOL IN CORK

Though London hosted dental hospitals from 1839, Birmingham pioneered formal dental training in Britain and Ireland. A dental hospital was founded in 1858 at (what became) the University of Birmingham, with formal training of dental students beginning in 1880. By 1900 the school was awarding the new dental degree, the Bachelor of Dental Surgery (BDS).

In Dublin, a dental hospital opened in 1879, and the Irish branch of the British Dental Association was formed the following year. The Royal College of Surgeons in Ireland awarded its first LDS in 1884. In 1904 the University of Dublin (now UCD) began offering dental degrees and diplomas, with Trinity College Dublin (TCD) following in 1910. The Dublin dental hospital provided the primary dental professional credential used in Ireland. Ultimately, the hospital hosted students engaged in three separate BDS and LDS degree programmes at UCD, TCD and the Royal College of Surgeons in Ireland.

In Cork, an 1844 commercial directory shows eight dentists practising in the city centre. That number stayed relatively constant during the ensuing decades. By 1881 a dentist had been appointed to the Cork Ophthalmic and Aural Hospital, and ten years later the number of Cork dentists had risen to eleven. By the end of the century, those possessing LDS qualifications began to include them in their directory listings, calling themselves a 'registered dentist'. Professional dentistry was firmly established in Cork.

Meanwhile, 'up above' at University College Cork (UCC) serious change was afoot. The university had come under the leadership of Sir Bertram Windle, perhaps the most important president in UCC history. A professor of anatomy, Windle had been hired by UCC on the basis of his achievements as the University of Birmingham Medical School's first dean. In that role he collaborated closely with Birmingham's successful dental school and hospital. Windle helped the school become Britain's first university to award the BDS and MDS (Master of Dental Surgery) degrees. According to one observer, Windle 'held that the University Degrees could not fail to enhance the prestige of dentistry'. This experience likely inspired his later dental initiative at UCC.

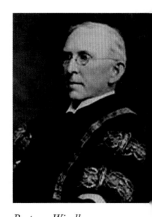

Bertram Windle, president of UCC.
Courtesy UCC Archive

Windle oversaw the transition from Queen's College Cork to the new National University of Ireland (NUI), University College Cork in 1909. However, he was not satisfied with Cork's NUI governance. Instead, he envisioned an independent Munster university, along the lines of Queen's University Belfast or the University of Birmingham. Over the next decade, the independent-Munster-university project consumed Windle. Beyond its practicalities, it reinforced his political loyalties as a supporter of Irish home rule and of John Redmond's Irish Party. To secure 'educational home rule' for Cork, Windle rapidly expanded the university.

In the next few years, Windle created a host of new professorships in archaeology, economics, education, German, Irish, mathematical physics, medical jurisprudence, music, ophthalmology, pathology and natural history. Student numbers climbed rapidly. In the previous fifteen years, the average first-year student entry was fifty students. During 1909–10, 102 first-year students entered UCC, a figure that grew to 181 in 1910–11. The student body increased from 171 in 1900–01 to 404 in 1910–11.

During this period of rapid growth, Windle decided to create a dental school. UCC had been closely associated with medicine since its foundation (a link retained in the college sports teams' current skull-and-crossbones emblem). This legacy predated the university, reaching back to the Cork Anatomy School opened in 1811. A new dental school would strengthen Cork's medical faculty and bolster the independent-Munster-university initiative.

Windle asked the city's small community of credentialed dentists to create a university-affiliated dental school and hospital. Twelve of fourteen registered dentists in Cork joined the dental hospital as honorary staff, essentially running the school without pay. Hubert O'Keeffe, a registered dentist, was appointed the first dean. The other founding members were all local registered dentists in private practice: P.B. Birmingham, Louis Egan, William Gates, James Hackett, Thomas Ollivere, Stanley Sullivan, William Pericho, F.M.H. Sanderson, Israel Scher, George Sheedy and Arthur Wiley. Many were trying to build their own careers, with six having registered as dentists within the previous five years. Available census information indicates that six were Catholic, four Church of Ireland and one Jewish (the other's religious affiliation could not be ascertained). These founding fathers of the Cork University Dental School and Hospital seemed to have intended to strengthen dentistry in Cork as a scientific, ethical and respectable profession.

On 7 March 1913 the UCC Medical Faculty approved the degree of Bachelor in Dental Surgery (BDS). Students would receive academic courses at UCC and clinical training at a newly established dental hospital. Two members of the hospital staff

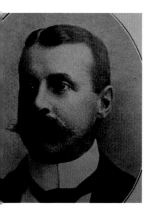

Hubert O'Keeffe,
the first dean of CUDSH.
Courtesy Peter O'Donoghue

were appointed to lectureships at UCC, which were part-time, unpaid positions. Student clinical instruction was carried out under the auspices of the publicly financed North Charitable Infirmary (commonly called the 'North Infirmary' or the 'North Cha') located in the impoverished Shandon neighbourhood on the city's north side. At that time, the hospital had 109 beds and was one of the largest in Cork. Bertram Windle explained the rationale for locating the dental hospital in a severely deprived area of Cork city:

> It is true that there are dental surgeons of ability attached to several Cork Hospitals but up to the present no provision has been made for any other treatment of the teeth than that of extractions. Now, as everyone knows, the extraction of the teeth nowadays is but a small part of the treatment available for a dentist. Conservative Dentistry, so called, has made enormous strides since the Dental profession was properly constituted. There has, however, been no provision made to enable the poorer classes of Cork to profit by such treatment, though it was and is available for those who can afford to pay the ordinary fees of the qualified Dental Surgeon. This was in no way the fault or desire of the Dental practitioners as shown by the readiness they welcomed the suggestion of a Dental Hospital and placed their services fully, freely and gratuitously at its disposal to their great credit.

In the first months of the school's existence, clinical students worked in what became the boardroom of the North Infirmary. Shortly thereafter, the dental hospital moved across the road to a building on Mulgrave Road (now John Redmond Street). The North Infirmary had acquired a converted butter warehouse (a relic of Cork's former global butter trade) that housed the Extern

Patient Department. A dental hospital was created on the first floor of that premises, though it had to make do with only about sixteen hundred square feet of space. The structure was leased from Edward Neville for £40 per annum on a healthy three-hundred-year lease. The dental hospital and the North Infirmary split the rent evenly, leaving CUDSH with a manageable operating cost.

J.R. Hackett and George Sheedy secured the prestigious, if unpaid, UCC lecturing posts in dental surgery and dental mechanics respectfully. Additional teaching responsibilities were delegated to hospital lecturers: P.B. Birmingham (dental surgery and pathology), George Sheedy (dental mechanics), A.C. Wiley (dental materia medica), Israel Scher (orthodontia) and T.S. Sullivan (dental anatomy). The only salaried staff members were the two non-dentists: dental mechanic G.L. Palmer and the hospital matron, Sr Josephine. The latter came from the Sisters of Charity of St Vincent de Paul (known simply as the Sisters of Charity), a religious order that provided trained nurses to the North Infirmary. Nuns from the order acted as the dental-hospital matron (manager) until the 1960s. An additional staff member joined the staff in 1914: Tom C. Butterfield, a leader of John Redmond's Irish Party in Cork. Butterfield seems to have been appointed primarily for his political connections, as he rarely attended the hospital during his ten-year service.

The initial degree-course structure was for a first year of pre-dental, consisting of physics, chemistry and anatomy; a second year consisting of anatomy, physiology and histology; a third year consisting of pathology, surgery, medicine, dental surgery, dental mechanics, dental-hospital mechanics and anaesthetics; and a fourth year consisting of dental mechanics, dental surgery, dental-hospital practice, orthodontia and dental materia medica. A fifth year was added in the 1940s. For many lectures, students commuted from the dental hospital to the university. Because of the part-time status of the twelve CUDSH staff, students attended some lectures in the waiting room of their teachers' private practices, seven of which were located in the South Mall, Cork.

The school admitted its first students in 1913, and awarded the first degrees in 1915. The recipients were William Foley and Eugene Whelan. Two years later, Mary O'Connor became the first woman to receive a BDS at CUDSH. Some early students were established dentists seeking an LDS so they could join the dental registry.

In 1914 the Cork dental hospital secured its own stationary, with a distinct masthead and Latin motto: 'Sanara sane divinum meliusque esi arcere quam mederi'; this can be freely translated as 'Prevention is better than cure'. To certain readers one hundred years later, this message retains an enduring appeal.

WAR & REVOLUTION

The foundation of Cork University Dental School and Hospital coincided with one of the most turbulent periods in modern Irish history. At the time of the opening of the dental hospital, Ireland was still governed as part of the United Kingdom. Within a year, a world war began that would change local political allegiances. It produced a decade of turmoil, which included a revolution and a civil war that divided the community.

Politics rarely directly penetrated the safety of UCC and CUDSH. Their avoidance by the hospital administration is not surprising considering the mixed unionist and nationalist identities of staff members. However, the war and political situation created an environment that implicitly affected the school and hospital. Among UCC's then current and former staff and students, thirty-nine died in the conflict, while nearly four hundred served with the British forces. In common with the practice in other academic departments, the dental school gifted two months' extra credit to Ernest O'Shea so that he could secure his degree and join the

THOMAS C. BUTTERFIELD:
THE BEST-ARMED DENTIST IN EUROPE

The Cork University Dental School and Hospital made a cameo appearance in the national drama known as the Easter Rising through the services of part-time staff member Thomas C. Butterfield. Born in 1863, 'Tackie' Butterfield qualified as an LDS and opened a practice on the South Mall. A noted athlete, he later served as president of the Munster branch of the Irish Rugby Football Union, and was a standout rower at Shandon Rowing Club. At the turn of the century, Butterfield emerged as a prominent political operator within John Redmond's Irish Party in Cork. Elected to Cork Corporation, he rose to become lord mayor in 1916.

Butterfield had only been lord mayor a few months when the Easter Rising broke out. Confusion reigned at the outset of the rebellion, as Cork's Irish Volunteers received conflicting orders from two opposing republican leadership groups in Dublin. The Patrick Pearse faction appealed to the Cork Volunteers to initiate combat operations in support of the Rising. However, Eoin MacNeill, the national commander of the Irish Volunteers, ordered Cork to stand down. Unclear of the situation in Dublin, the Cork commanders Tomás MacCurtain and Terence MacSwiney barricaded themselves and about a hundred armed men inside their hall on Sheares Street, ready to resist any government efforts to disarm them. The British army garrison at Victoria Barracks (now Collins Barracks) threatened to storm the Volunteer headquarters, which would have brought destructive fighting into the city centre.

Lord Mayor Butterfield and the Catholic bishop Daniel Cohalan appealed to the Irish Volunteers and British army officials to avoid any provocative actions that would initiate hostilities. As the standoff dragged on for days, Butterfield and Bishop Cohalan shuttled between Sheares Street and Victoria Barracks.

Their diplomacy ultimately secured a compromise over the status of the Volunteers' arms. MacCurtain and MacSwiney agreed to temporarily surrender their weapons to a neutral third party, Lord Mayor Butterfield, with the understanding that he would return them after the crisis passed.

On the Saturday after Easter Monday, about one hundred Irish Volunteers proceeded to Butterfield's dental practice on the South Mall and turned over seventy-five rifles and shotguns. However, not all the republicans agreed with the decision. Some surrendered wooden rifles used for drilling, passing their real weapons to Cumann na mBan members to be smuggled to safety. One enterprising Volunteer dropped off a fake rifle but palmed Butterfield's functioning pistol, which he kept in his office desk.

Butterfield's reign as the best-armed dentist in Europe did not last long. After the Dublin rebels surrendered, the British army seized the weapons stored in Butterfield's office. As public opinion shifted towards the new independence movement, Butterfield's political star sank with that of his party leader John Redmond. Though asked, he refused to stand in the 1918 general election, and in 1919 retired from public life. He continued in private practice and remained affiliated to CUDSH until the mid-1920s. He died in 1935. Butterfield's practice, however, stayed in the family, so to speak. Joe Power (BDS 1952), a CUDSH instructor from 1954 to 1963, purchased the practice upon his return from England. Butterfield's old practice has carried on through Joe's son Aidan Power (BDS 1993), maintaining the dental school's link to the dental arsenal.

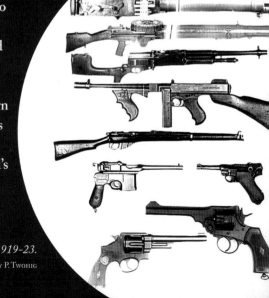

Irish republican weapons, 1919–23.
Courtesy P. Twohig

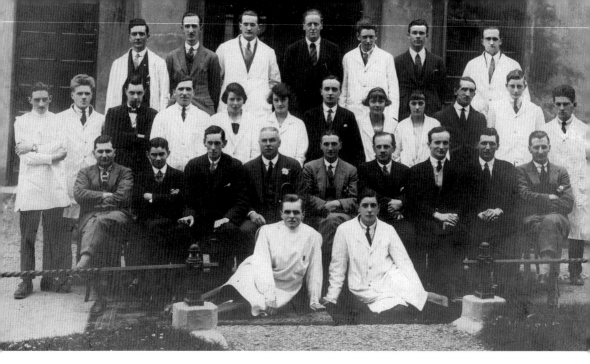

Cork Dental Hospital,
1922–23: (back, left to right)
A. Mahoney, R.F. Twomey,
J. O'Driscoll, M.J. Hunt,
F. Ferguson, J.L. Monaghan,
J.A. O'Mahony;
(centre, left to right)
R.L. Gallagher, T. Murphy,
J.J. Kelleher, P. O'Riordan,
Miss Pomeroy,
Miss Quinlan,
R. Vincent Ward,
Miss Goggin, Miss Clarke,
J.F. Hayes, N. Kearney,
J.A. O'Sullivan;
(front, left to right)
S.J. Morrough,
L.C. O'Mahony, G. Sheedy,
H. O'Keeffe, W.V. Pericho,
I. Scher, D.J. O'Mahony,
E. Murphy, C. Donfoy;
(sitting on ground, left to
right) F. Shanahan,
J. O'Meara.
COURTESY BRIAN O'RIORDAN

Royal Navy. Another student broke off his studies to enlist in the British military.

During these same years, a revolution broke out in Ireland. By mid-1920 Cork city had become a centre of guerrilla warfare against Crown forces. Shootings and bombings occurred close to the dental hospital, while the North Infirmary frequently treated casualties. The Shandon neighbourhood overlooked the city centre, and gunfire created a distinct echo in its narrow streets. In 1921 Irish Republican Army (IRA) fighters subjected the nearby Shandon Royal Irish Constabulary barracks to bomb and gun attacks. During 1922 republicans constructed armoured cars in a mechanic's premises on Leitrim Street, just below the large windows in the hospital conservation room. Civil-war sniping and bombing attacks continued in the area during 1922 and 1923.

It is unclear if any of the dental students participated in revolutionary activity, though it loomed in the background of student and faculty life in this period. Staff member Louis Egan came from a prominent republican family (his brother was the Sinn Féin deputy lord mayor), and his father's jewellery shop was deliberately burned by Crown forces in December 1920. The IRA apparently attempted to assassinate school co-founder James Hackett after he was mistaken for his brother, an outspoken anti-republican naval officer. A number of prominent IRA Volunteers were UCC medical students, and would have been known to dental students. Most UCC students attended the funerals of two members of the student body who died on IRA service in 1920 and 1921 (Christopher Lucey, killed at Ballingeary, and John Joe Joyce, killed at Clonmult). In November 1920, following the death of Terence MacSwiney whilst on hunger strike, university staff and students stood as a body on the Western Road to pay homage to the lord mayor's passing funeral cortège. The university adjoined Cork men's prison, which was filled with republican prisoners from 1917 to 1923. Frequent prisoner uprisings, hunger strikes and occasional attempted escapes created disturbances that were often audible and visible to those attending lectures on campus.

CUDSH seemed to have largely ignored the bloodshed erupting around it during these years. Weeks after Crown forces burned Cork city centre, dental students issued a public protest … against new legislation that grandfathered non-qualified dental practitioners onto the dental register. The Cork public intensely followed Dáil Éireann's ratification of the Anglo-Irish Treaty in January 1922, which established the new Irish Free State. The dental-hospital staff responded to the event by promptly appealing to the new Provisional Government to address the problem of unregistered dentists. The dental-hospital staff-meeting minutes do not mention the devastating Irish civil war, except to protest about the non-payment for treatment of National Army troops at the hospital and the military's failure to form a proper dental corps. Hospital staff and dental students must have quietly acknowledged the political conflict engulfing the country, though they rarely directly engaged with it.

The conflict wreaked havoc on public finances in the country. Residents paid roughly half the local taxes due from 1919 to 1922, inspired by both political and mercenary reasons. Infrastructure and public buildings suffered badly in various rounds of fighting between the Crown forces, the IRA and the National Army. About ninety shops were destroyed during the 'burning of Cork' by police in December 1920. A post-war recession also hit the country, shutting businesses and driving up unemployment. The new Irish Free State, burdened with the cost of the civil war, was essentially broke by 1923. This meant it was an extremely difficult period in which to launch a new medical-education and health-care-service institution. CUDSH was further handicapped by the loss of a strong supporter, President Betram Windle. Unsuccessful in his effort to secure an independent Munster university and wary of the chaotic political situation, he departed UCC in 1919.

Within a few short years, the dental hospital would find itself operating under a government with few funds and little interest in public health. Born into war and revolution and soon orphaned, the school entered adolescence struggling to survive as a permanent medical-education institution.

2

EARLY YEARS

----

*T*HOUGH handicapped by a poor economy, unsettled national politics and an impoverished government, the Cork University Dental School and Hospital consolidated its gains and established itself as a centre of dental education. The process was slow, and was undertaken through a series of baby steps in the ensuing years.

COURSE OF STUDY

During the school's first decade, enrolment usually averaged between two and five students annually. Students received instruction from 9 am to 5 pm, Monday to Friday, plus a Saturday half-day session (9 am to 1 pm). Clinical work took place at the hospital during the morning, after which students crossed town to attend medical lectures at UCC. Those lectures were usually delivered by part-time teachers who travelled to college from local hospitals or their private practices, and there were often significant delays. Waiting students frequently gathered in the Men's Club until summoned to class by a bell. The university's total student body was under a thousand in these years, so dental students were integrated into college life despite spending considerable time off campus. Dental and medical students often developed close friendships, since they shared numerous classes in their first and second years. Classroom instruction was also provided at UCC by two honorary dentistry lecturers, who were part-time and essentially unpaid. Additional courses were offered at the dental hospital by the part-time teaching staff.

When students did not have afternoon lectures at UCC, they were instructed in practical dental mechanics (making impression trays, dentures, crowns and so on) at the hospital. This training was needed because dental mechanics were often in short supply, while dental nursing was unknown at this time. The mechanical emphasis enabled Cork graduates to operate essentially as one-man-bands when needed, which bolstered their employment options after qualification.

Students progressed after passing end-of-year subject exams. UCC courses (those offered at the university campus rather than the dental hospital) featured external examiners, who were often dental educators from the United Kingdom. However, course exams held at the dental hospital do not appear to have used externs until the mid-1950s. This reflects an institutional informality more in synch with the old dental apprenticeship system than modern medical education. Along the same lines, some students from the 1950s and 1960s recall instructors occasionally hiding or obscuring their own personal treatment techniques lest they be 'stolen' by a future competitor (the student).

Dental-hospital conditions appear to have been fairly spartan. There was no canteen and no cloakroom until 1956. There may have been little need for the latter as photographs show students in the hospital wearing overcoats, which would indicate a cold building (coal being a major operating cost). The school began a paltry library in 1919, based on a small gift from Dean Hubert O'Keeffe. The North Infirmary board of management made a one-time grant of £10 towards the purchase of books, and a second grant of £20 followed a mere fourteen years later. In the ensuing decades, staff periodically made small contributions towards the purchase of new texts, or donated their own professional journals for student use. However, the poor library remained a concern until the early 1990s.

Though student facilities were limited, student regulations became formalised in late 1919. The staff adopted a series of rules for student conduct, which required the precise recording of attendance and practice work. The new rules read:

1. That cards be given every month to students – to show a record of their attendance and work completed.

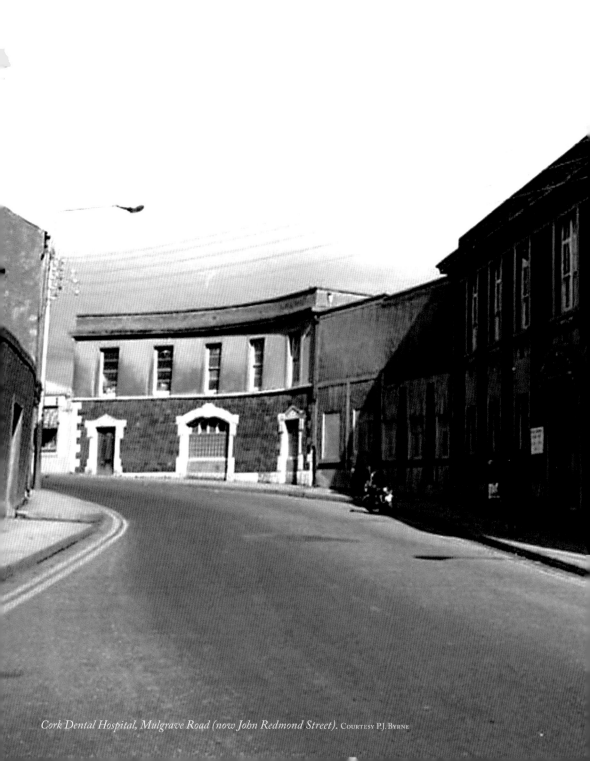

Cork Dental Hospital, Mulgrave Road (now John Redmond Street). Courtesy P.J. Byrne

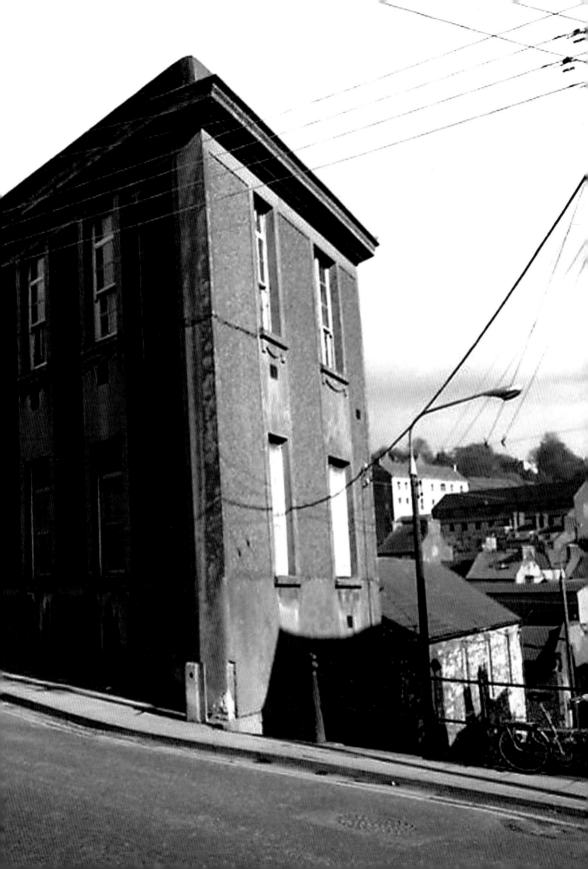

2. Leave of absence must be obtained through the Dean of the Hospital. If a student is unable to attend through sickness he must provide a medical certificate.
3. Attendance of students – students' roll to be closed at 9:15AM sharp.
4. If a student is late and cannot get a mark he loses a day.
5. Appointments made by students must be kept – penalty for not keeping them is lose a day.
6. All fillings and cavities to be signed by members of staff or house surgeons. No credit given for work done unless signed.
7. House surgeons to insist on making students use rubber dam whenever possible.
8. Students to supply their own gold for phantom heads.
9. Students to apply to House Surgeons for patients.
10. 'No smoking' in any part of the operating rooms.
11. Students' cabinets to be inspected monthly by the dean.

Small student numbers resulted in close learning relationships, as students received extensive personal attention. Clinical work required students to work shoulder to shoulder with staff, who provided encouragement to unsteady beginners.

SCHOOL & HOSPITAL OPERATIONS

The deanship changed a number of times in these early years. The school's first dean, Hubert O'Keeffe, was reportedly the first licensed dental surgeon (LDS) in Ireland, having qualified in 1881. However, he resigned for unknown reasons in 1919 and was succeeded by William Pericho, who had only qualified for an LDS in 1903. The son of a tramway-company clerk of Italian extraction, Pericho, like many later faculty members, was popularly remembered as a devoted golfer. Pericho's eleven-year reign was abruptly ended by his unexpected death at the age of forty-five.

His successor, George Sheedy, had been a co-founder of the Cork dental hospital, and had qualified in 1912. Unfortunately, as with his predecessor, Sheedy's tenure was also ended by his premature death, in 1932.

By this stage the Cork dental school had suffered an alarming drop in enrolment. Measured by BDS graduates, CUDSH began slowly, qualifying only four students in its first three years. However, numbers gradually rose thereafter. By 1918, graduates increased to six, and 1925 produced an unprecedented nine degrees. Overall, from 1918 to 1928 the school graduated an average of four students per year. However, student numbers began to drop in 1929, as the Great Depression took hold in Ireland. Enrolment declined from four in 1928 to one in 1929, before the barren years of 1930, 1931 and 1932, when no students qualified.

At this stage Israel Scher took over the deanship. A Cork native educated at Presentation College, he qualified from the Royal College of Surgeons with first-class honours in 1909. A co-founder of the school, Scher provided steady leadership during his sixteen-year tenure as dean. It was a difficult period for the school, which faced major national crises with the Economic War and the Second World War. Beyond keeping CUDSH on an even keel, Scher also brought an academic emphasis that slowly steered the school away from the dental-apprenticeship system.

The dean's role was to administer policy decisions made collectively by the dental-school staff. Eventually, the voluntary faculty divided into senior and junior levels, with the senior staff given voting rights. In these early years, the hospital faculty occasionally acted to maintain standards of the local dental profession. In 1917 the staff complained to the British Dental Association about a dental practitioner who left calling cards in hotel waiting rooms and posted an 'unduly large' name plate. A few years later, a special hospital delegation visited Dáil Éireann to lobby for the regulation of advertisements by dental surgeons. Ultimately, such professional

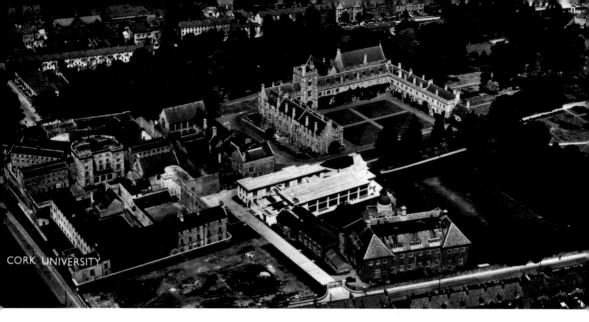

CORK UNIVERSITY

*University College Cork.
campus.* Courtesy UCC Archives

responsibilities were assumed by what became the Munster branch of the Irish Dental Association (IDA) (which seems to have come into being around 1932). In these early decades, the broader professionalisation of dentistry can be seen in the actions of CUDSH staff.

The dental school operated its off-campus hospital with little input from University College Cork. The departure of the UCC president Bertram Windle in 1919 left the dental school without a powerful institutional advocate. In the following decades, Windle's successors rarely engaged with CUDSH except when it faced existential problems or threatened to embarrass the parent university (or both). Similarly, CUDSH and the UCC School of Medicine rarely interacted, a remoteness that continued until relatively recently. Members of the dental-school staff in more recent decades have described a long-standing inferiority complex felt by dental students and lecturers vis-à-vis the medical faculty. One graduate recalled, 'we thought of ourselves as a poor relation', a sentiment not entirely of their own creation. For many of the dental-school's staff and students, as far as UCC was concerned they remained both out of sight and out of mind.

While CUDSH was situated in close physical proximity to the North Infirmary, relations were seldom better than those with

UCC, at least in the school's first decade. The North Infirmary governing body administered the dental hospital, maintaining control over budgets, personnel, purchases and major policy matters. However, the governing body contained no CUDSH representative, which left the latter without a voice regarding hospital policy that affected it. This contributed to a dysfunctional relationship, which was compounded by the staff's lack of full-time positions or payment of its volunteer teachers, a condition about which members frequently complained. Fire was not one-way. In 1927, for example, after the governing body failed to force an appointment onto the dental faculty, a board member claimed some dental-school staff members were 'more ornamental than useful'. Two disputes occurring twenty years apart illustrated long-standing tensions within Irish medical administration: the reluctance to pay for public medical services and the role of the Catholic Church in medical treatment.

TENSIONS

In 1923 the governing body convinced a reluctant dental hospital to accept any patient with national health insurance and to treat schoolchildren. However, the dental-school staff rejected the North Infirmary's proposal for the dental hospital to care for nearly thirteen thousand Cork schoolchildren in a scheme paid for by Cork Corporation. Such large-scale treatment was simply not feasible with the part-time staff available; it would also (presumably) eat into their own private practices. At the end of 1924, the staff likewise refused the North Infirmary's request to open the dental hospital in the evening (from 7–9 pm) twice a week, since no overtime payments were provided to attending staff.

Undeterred, in June 1925 the North Infirmary governing body instructed the dental-school staff to treat thousands of Cork schoolchildren annually at the dental hospital. Like many of the new

Irish state's public-health initiatives, the programme was woefully underfunded and reliant on semi-charitable institutions. It also set to boil a pot that had been simmering for the previous two years.

The dental-school staff determined that the proposed scheme required at least one full-time school dentist. The governing body proceeded to advertise for this new position, at the low annual salary of £150. The staff strongly objected to the 'totally inadequate' pay rate, which it believed would diminish 'the state of the profession'. The governing body increased the salary to £350, to be divided by two part-time dentists. Thus, two half-time positions were created, which the dental-hospital staff still considered insufficient. Having been ignored throughout the planning process, the hospital staff threatened to resign as a body if the governing body proceeded with the appointment. Undeterred, the governing body set about filling the two posts in the first week of September 1925. The staff duly notified the governing body that they were resigning on the eighth of the month, 'to uphold the dignity of our profession'. Members pointed out that:

- They were unpaid;
- They had no voice on the North Infirmary governing body administering the dental hospital;
- The governing body was unwilling to create an adequately paid, full-time position, which showed a fundamental lack of respect for the dental profession.

Beyond the protest over the filling of the school-dentist position, staff members remained upset at the lack of consultation with them regarding the decision to open the dental hospital in the evenings. At the heart of the dispute was the dental hospital's continued absence on the North Infirmary governing body, in contrast to the represented North Infirmary medical staff. To the dental-hospital staff, the denial of a voice in matters pertaining to its operations reflected the North Infirmary's unequal treatment of dentistry compared with medicine.

As the dispute escalated, the governing body expressed dismay at the dental-school staff's 'undignified' stance. One member complained that 'if the staff were to run the hospital in their own way the Committee had better resign', while another blustered that 'this has always been their cry, and we ought to have had enough of it'. Another even suggested they 'close up the place altogether, and we could open it afterwards under more satisfactory conditions'. However, cooler heads voted against filling the new vacancy, thus delaying a decision until after the board met with the dental-hospital staff. The governing body lacked any real leverage since the dental faculty was unpaid and virtually irreplaceable, owing to the fact that it contained virtually every qualified dentist in Cork.

The dental-school staff informed the governing body that they would parley in early October, after some faculty members had returned from holiday. On Friday 11 September, the teaching staff did not appear for their rotations, forcing the governing body to close the hospital until further notice. The strike occurred just prior to student registration for the new academic year, which risked the institution's future. Concerned that the situation was getting out of hand, North Infirmary and dental-hospital officials huddled over the weekend to find a resolution. On Monday the dental-school staff agreed to operate the hospital on a reduced schedule until early October. When the staff reconvened a few weeks later, they accepted the governing body's appointment. The governing body promptly co-opted Dean Israel Scher as a new member, thus giving the dental hospital a clear vote in its governance. The compromise seemed to satisfy both sides. Meanwhile, two part-time school dentists worked at the hospital on alternate afternoons. This arrangement continued until 1938, when Cork Corporation opened a school dental clinic in the City Hall.

One of the new school dentists was Helen Goggin, who had

Like other military conflicts, the First World War produced major advances in medicine in such areas as prosthetics, skin grafts and trauma-surgery techniques. The war also brought about improved dentistry, mainly in reconstructive surgery (treating mouth wounds) and in the mass introduction of dental treatment to ordinary working people. With the creation of enormous conscription armies, the British army needed dentists, which led to the establishment of the Royal Army Dental Corps (RADC) in 1921. This new military medical branch offered job security to Irish dentists willing to serve in the British army after Irish independence. Remarkably, two Cork graduates headed the RADC in the post-Second World War period. Both received the unique distinction of serving as honorary dental surgeon to the reigning British monarch.

Corkman John Wren (BDS 1918) was one of Cork's first graduates, qualifying five years before his brother William. Wren was educated at Christian Brothers College (Cork), and lived at Flanagan's Hotel in Winthrop Street, operated by his father, a retired Customs and Excise official. Joining the Royal Air Force after graduation, he quickly transferred to the British army. He rose steadily through the RADC ranks, ultimately becoming its commanding major-general. From this position, he acted as dental surgeon to George VI. Wren was awarded a CBE, and attended Elizabeth II's coronation in 1953. Retiring in Surrey, he maintained links with the Irish Dental Association until his death a few years later.

Henry Quinlan (BDS 1926) enjoyed a strong connection with CUDSH through his sister Denise (BDS 1925). A female teaching pioneer in the school, she later married Ned Murphy, a long-time and much beloved staff member. The Quinlans hailed from Fermoy, and their father was a doctor whose practice included the local British army barracks. Joining the RADC as a lieutenant in 1927, Henry served overseas in Hong Kong and Shanghai. During the Second World War, he successfully evacuated his mobile dental unit from France after the fall of Dunkirk in 1940. Finishing the war in India, he helped establish the Pakistani Dental Corps, which was led by one of his subordinates immediately after independence. After his return to England, Henry was appointed honorary dental surgeon to the queen in 1954, and served in that position until his retirement in 1963. Like John Wren, he was appointed director of the RADC with the rank of major-general in 1958, and was also awarded a CBE. Quinlan served as colonel-commandant of the RADC until his retirement in 1969. In later years, he continued in military dentistry, taking up civilian positions at the Supreme Headquarters Allied Powers Europe in Paris and, finally, at the Guards Depot in Pirbright, Surrey. He died in 2000, at the age of 94.

Major-General Henry Quinlan, CB.
Courtesy Royal Army Dental Corps Archive

The rise of two Cork graduates to the pinnacle of British-military dentistry testifies to the high quality of graduates produced by CUDSH, even in difficult times. Their careers showed that, when given the opportunity, Cork alumni could successfully compete with anyone in Britain and Ireland.

been the first women to serve on the dental-hospital staff. She was succeeded by another female Cork graduate, Denise Quinlan. The experience of these two teaching pioneers reflected a contradiction apparent among female Irish professionals in this period. While women could obtain university qualifications, their subsequent careers were often constrained by gender expectations. They were expected to resign their posts when they married, and were frequently pigeonholed into positions related to their gender. Indeed, both Helen Goggin and Denise Quinlan were hired to consult on the dental treatment of children, a maternal role still considered at that time to be 'women's work'. (Quinlan retained a lifelong affiliation with the dental school through her husband Edward 'Ned' Murphy, a popular member of the teaching staff.)

Another gender-designated role in the dental hospital was that of matron. At CUDSH, Catholic nuns from the Sisters of Charity filled that position until the 1960s. Their presence occasionally created difficulties for hospital officials negotiating Church–state relations in the devout Irish state, as seen in the Sr Brendan episode. In 1946 the dental-school staff sought, for unknown reasons (almost certainly performance-related), to dismiss Sr Brendan after six years' service as hospital matron. Staff members seemed reluctant to raise the matter publicly and risk a possible public backlash. Instead, they approached the UCC president, Alfred O'Rahilly, a devout Catholic often perceived as excessively deferential to the clergy. President O'Rahilly and staff member Michael Roche visited Revd Mother Raphael, head of the Sisters of Charity order attached to the North Infirmary. According to O'Rahilly, 'I made it quite clear that our interview was confidential and we were dealing with Mother Raphael in her capacity as Religious Superior'. As such, they asked the mother superior for a change in personnel, which was agreed to.

Despite their caution, the North Infirmary governing body caught wind of Sr Brendan's removal, and added it to the agenda

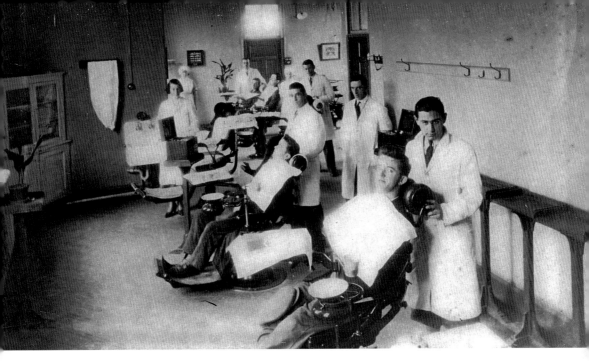

for its next meeting, which was printed in the *Cork Examiner*. A horrified O'Rahilly informed the governing body that such open discussion was 'a gross breach of good taste and a piece of unpleasant and gratuitous publicity' that might embarrass the Sisters of Charity. The governing body in turn asked why the dental hospital made such an important decision without prior consultation. O'Rahilly and the hospital staff replied with public statements explaining that Sr Brendan's replacement was an internal matter for the Sisters of Charity, 'who presumably claim the right to transfer their subjects without obtaining the permission of a lay board'. The explanation satisfied the governing body, which appeared unwilling to engage in a public controversy with a religious body. Such caution was entirely consistent with Church–state relations during this period of Irish history. Not surprisingly, the Jewish school dean, Israel Scher, distanced himself from the removal decision (arousing anger among staff members), and seems to have deliberately assigned a Catholic member of the dental-school staff (Michael Roche) to accompany President O'Rahilly on his mission. For Scher, discretion was the better part of valour, at least in cases entailing possible clashes with the Catholic Church.

Main conservation room, old dental hospital, 1930/31: CUDSH historian Ray Gamble stands behind the centre dental chair with patient, while teaching pioneer Denise Quinlan stands to his right in front of the basin.
Courtesy UCC Archives

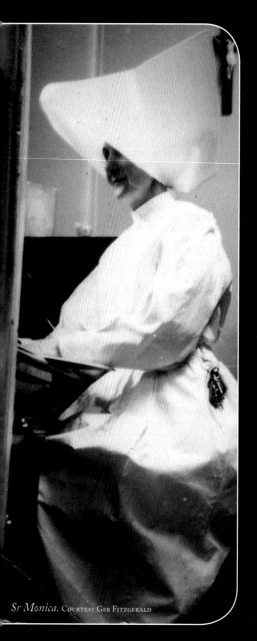

Sr Monica. COURTESY GER FITZGERALD

Modern observers often note the distinctive presence of a nun's winged habit while viewing old photographs of the dental-hospital staff. Indeed, until the 1960s members of the Sisters of Charity religious order filled the position of hospital matron. These devoted nuns were fixtures in the first dental hospital on John Redmond Street.

The Sisters of Charity in Cork were members of the Irish province of the Daughters of Charity of St Vincent de Paul. The French order served the poor, and first came to Ireland in 1855 following the Famine. Within a few years, the order had attached itself to Cork's North Infirmary Charitable Hospital, which cared for the city's most impoverished residents. The sisters worked as nurses and administrators in the North Infirmary, and lived in a small residence adjoining the 'North Cha'.

Once the dental hospital was founded, a Sister of Charity was appointed matron in 1914. The sister in charge acted as the hospital operations manager, assuming responsibility for purchasing, accounting and supply inventories. The matron also interviewed first-time patients to ascertain their financial status, which determined whether or not they would be charged for treatment. Essentially, the matron saw to tasks large and small that kept the hospital running smoothly.

One of the best-remembered hospital

matrons was Sr Monica, who served the dental hospital from 1949 to 1969. Born Mary McCarthy, she had qualified in medicine at UCC before entering the Sisters of Charity. She was remembered as a 'wonderful administrator' who was also 'very thrifty'. Her frugality suited well a dental hospital surviving on a tight financial margin. 'She almost measured the filling material by the grains', remembered long-time staff member Theresa O'Mahony.

Sr Monica also took a keen interest in the welfare of students, checking in with individuals periodically and monitoring their health and progress. Her tenure overlapped with a great expansion of the student body, and she ensured that none of them were lost in the shuffle.

Alumni from this era commonly associate Sr Monica with the rosary. At the end of the school day, Sr Monica gathered up students to kneel and say a decade of the rosary. It was alleged that she would occasionally ask students to pray for the conversion of non-Catholics on the hospital staff, including the Scher brothers. However, she was tactful enough to do so when they were not present in the hospital. Such piety reflected Ireland's intense Catholicism during this period, though it should not be overstated. In terms of Sr Monica's rosary, Cork graduates also recalled certain irreverent students kneeling behind the good sister and having contests to see who could toss the most plaster of Paris chips into her habit. Sr Monica appeared blissfully unaware of her habit's dual role as basketball hoop.

The Sisters of Charity did not follow the dental school into its new hospital in Wilton. If their devoutness has become less common in Irish society, the nuns' administrative skills and good sense remain valued commodities to any institution. The following Sisters of Charity should be remembered for their service as matrons of the Cork dental hospital: Sr Theresa (1914–19), Sr Vincent (1920), Sr Josephine (1921–30), Sr Ann (1931–39), Sr Brendan (1940–46) and Sr Monica (1949–69).

FINANCES

The matron position remained critical owing to CUDSH's tight operating budget. Largely self-funded, the hospital survived on very narrow margins. A stream of paying patients generated enough income to cover supplies and building maintenance, while technical services at the hospital provided revenue from dentists in private practice. Yet it was a precarious existence. Describing the hospital as 'charitable rather than semi-charitable', one staff member wrote that fees frequently went unpaid. Expensive equipment required periodic replacement, which created major problems. Fortunately, at this stage relief came from the controversial Irish Hospital Sweepstakes.

Starting in 1930, the 'Irish Sweeps' funded cash-starved charity hospitals in Ireland by way of a lottery-style system, with the winning number determined by the results of selected horse races. Tickets sold (often illegally) among the Irish diaspora in Britain and the United States brought millions into the Irish health sector, making a number of shadowy Sweeps' operatives very wealthy in the process. The Irish Sweeps generated critical cash for the Cork dental hospital during the lean years of the Great Depression. The 1931 and 1933 drawings allocated a total of at least £10,000 to the dental hospital, providing much-welcomed financial breathing room.

CUDSH rested on firmer ground by the end of the decade. The 1938 annual hospital report recorded a healthy operating profit of £403 from a total budget of £10,928. Patient visits for the year totalled 8,779. Staff carried out 107 X-rays, 908 fillings and a remarkable 13,126 extractions, which reflected the preferred form of treatment. The Sweeps grants seemed to have been used to replace antiquated chairs in the conservation room, which were now twenty-five years old. The hospital bought six Berger chairs and new spittoons in 1938, despite Dean Scher's objections to purchasing the equipment from Nazi Germany. An architect was also commissioned to design a new hospital on the current site. However, the North Infirmary governing body rejected the construction plans. The dental-school staff would ultimately remain within its cramped confines for another forty-five years.

THE EMERGENCY & ITS IMPACT

Israel Scher's concerns about Hitler's Germany do not seem to have been shared by his colleagues. Similar to the dental-hospital's experience during the First World War and the Irish Revolution, CUDSH records rarely mention the global conflagration that raged between 1939 and 1945. The Irish government had declared a state of emergency at the outset of the war, but the reality of the situation only became apparent in June 1940 when France fell to Germany and the British army fled Dunkirk. Days after the Allied defeat, the dental faculty met to consider 'the duties of the staff in the state of National Emergency'. When the Battle of Britain erupted a few weeks later and made the invasion of Ireland seem increasingly likely, the staff started lecturing students on first aid, including bandaging and treating fractures. However, once the immediate crisis passed, the hospital largely returned to normal. The only major impact, according to dental-hospital historian Ray Gamble, was the shortage of porcelain (also experienced in Britain), which resulted in the increased use of plastics in the manufacture of teeth bases and denture bases.

The Second World War's greatest effect on Cork University Dental School and Hospital concerned Britain's plans to provide free health care to its citizens. Recommendations in the 1942 *Beveridge Report* eventually led to the creation of the National Health Service (NHS) in 1946. As a result, British citizens received free dental treatment, generating a massive demand for dentists. In Cork, the new situation dramatically altered student enrolment. Recognising lucrative employment possibilities, twelve

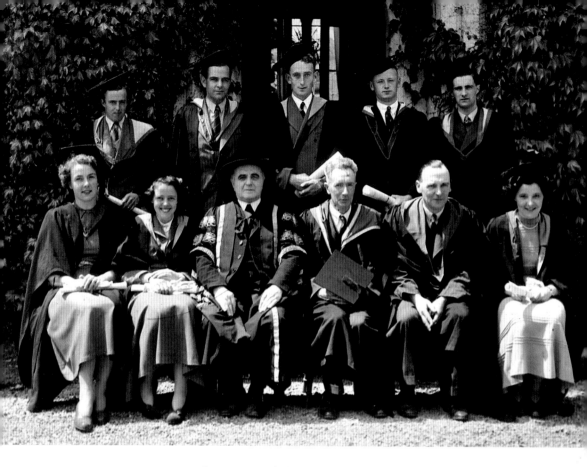

*BDS class of 1948:
(front, left to right)
M. Keating, M. Barry,
A. O'Rahilly, R. McConnell,
M. Roche, R. Gilleran;
(back, left to right)
P. O'Donoghue, J. Murray,
D. Gleeson, J. Markham,
W. Palmer.*
COURTESY WILLIE PALMER

new students entered the school in 1944, up from three in 1942. The school's days of one and two-person classes were over.

Almost overnight, dental education in Cork had changed significantly. A fresh set of challenges followed. CUDSH would need to keep pace with the rapid improvements in dental education experienced across Europe. The lack of proper public financing had to be resolved. Increased enrolment meant that new students had to be accommodated within the tiny hospital. Teaching could no longer be done by unpaid, part-time dental practitioners alone. These issues ultimately created a crisis for the Cork University Dental School and Hospital. Within two decades, the school would face a choice: modernise or perish.

3

MODERNISATION

THE introduction of the National Health Service in the United Kingdom transformed Irish dental education after the Second World War. The rapid expansion of British dental services created a demand for qualified dentists, which Irish dental schools happily helped fill. At CUDSH, student enrolment sky-rocketed, placing new pressures on the dental school and hospital. While British dental education enjoyed post-war increases in public investment, improved facilities and new staff hiring, Irish dental schools still operated with little state support. This ultimately led to unsatisfactory conditions that in 1961 nearly resulted in the closure of the Cork University Dental School and Hospital.

GROWTH

Cork graduation rates climbed steadily following the end of the Second World War. CUDSH produced an average of about two and a half graduates per year from 1940 to 1947. From 1950 to 1954 that number jumped to over eight annually, which was the maximum annual intake of students the hospital could then accommodate. Within seven years, annual student intake rose first to twelve, and then, in 1961, to sixteen.

Growth brought about changes in hospital facilities and in the education experience. The conservation room added new chairs, raising the total to ten. The rest of the surgical inventory included two dental engines, four spittoons, eight cabinet stands, seven tables and one nitrous-oxide gas apparatus. New students increased competition, which raised the prestige of annual prizes awarded by dental companies such as Panton & Company, the Dental Depot and Amalgamated Dental. (The annual prize-giving ceremony only began in the 1980s, but has become a key date in the school calendar under the direction of Claire O'Keeffe, a long-time and popular staff member.) Larger student classes also created an *esprit de corps* within CUDSH, making it a livelier and more enjoyable environment in which to study and work. This in turn necessitated a tightening of student discipline, as reflected in the banning of phone calls and smoking in the hospital. Indicative of the times, ten-minute smoke breaks were established in the morning and afternoon.

Higher student numbers did not necessarily improve the quality of Cork's BDS degree. Clinical work remained the school's primary strength. At a time when dental treatment remained out of reach for many Irish families, there was no shortage of patients. Impoverished city residents were 'wonderful people', one former student recalled, 'a cross between saints and martyrs'. As in previous decades, clinical work received the most attention, while dental theory and pathology were taught by self-educated part-time lecturers. Since the war, equipment and techniques had grown out of date, and some lecturers struggled to keep abreast of developments in their field. Former students from this period recall the revelation brought by their new part-time orthodontics lecturer, Rodney Dockrell, who later became dean of the TCD dental school: they were awed by a top-class lecturer who could both entertain and inform students. Dockrell was not the only effective lecturer at the Cork dental school, but there were other teachers who were undertrained, underqualified and reliant upon reading lessons from someone else's textbook. Students became aware of the strengths and limitations of their training.

EMIGRATION

Ireland's post-war economy languished and ultimately declined during the 1950s. Young people departed the country in massive numbers, depopulating many rural districts. With few job prospects at home and multiple opportunities in expanding economies abroad, a generation of young people left Ireland. A majority of emigrants relocated to the United Kingdom.

Ireland had already experienced mass relocations to Britain

during the Second World War to satisfy manpower shortages in British war industries. The movement continued so that by 1951 the Irish in Britain numbered nearly 700,000. Beyond the poor economic situation in Ireland, there were additional reasons for the outward flow to Britain. Irish people grew up exposed to British media, which created a comfortable cultural affinity. Britain was close to home physically and mentally, making eventual return to Ireland (often assumed by departing emigrants) seem more realistic.

Many recent arrivals came from poorer and undereducated segments of Irish society. In this period, two thirds of the population left school at the age of fourteen, and only about one out of a hundred completed university degrees. Irish dental emigrants constituted part of the national elite, and were, therefore, part of Ireland's 'brain drain' during the 1950s, as Irish university graduates and professionals departed for opportunities abroad, especially in Britain.

The level of emigration experienced by Cork graduates in the years after the Second World War seems extremely high, even in the context of the fiscal and youth unemployment crises then being experienced. Throughout the late 1940s and 1950s, waves of Cork-trained dentists left Ireland, primarily to England. By 1954 the new school dean, Jack Daunt, claimed eighty-five per cent of graduates were emigrating each year. In some cases, entire qualified classes from Cork left the country, such as the classes of 1962 and 1963. From 1960 to 1964, fifty-four of fifty-seven CUDSH graduates left Ireland, with fifty-three of them relocating to England. The dental exodus likely surpassed the departure of other Irish medical professionals, as historian Enda Delaney has estimated that between a quarter and a half of newly qualified Irish doctors were employed 'across the water' during these years. The disparity with medicine reflected the state of Irish dentistry at the time, which was poorly resourced privately and publicly, and thus offered few options for newly qualified dentists.

Cork graduates found high salaries in Britain, making it an

'El Dorado', as one graduate put it. After years of student poverty, 'fortunes were made overnight'. They purchased conspicuous sports cars and even their own homes – luxuries that seemed unattainable just a short time previously. Another former student remembered earning £100 per week at his first job in the UK. When he returned to Ireland a few years later to take up a position with the Irish public-health service, his weekly salary dropped to £27. Embracing an attitude to 'go over and make as much as we can', many CUDSH alumni found 'security, big money'.

Cork dental emigrants often linked into networks of recent graduates, as a form of professional 'chain migration'. Pockets of Cork dentists emerged in places such as Essex, Sussex, Kent, Brighton and North London. Unlike other Irish emigrants, the Cork dental graduates seemed to have integrated fairly easily since they frequently worked beyond the confines of the Irish community in Britain. Young, well-educated and upwardly mobile, they often joined established English dental practices that treated English patients. Though initially intimidated by their British-educated colleagues ('they had trained under the authors of our dental textbooks' explained one Cork graduate), Cork alumni found their abundant chair time put them in good standing. While undertrained with sophisticated dentistry such as crown work, they felt unsurpassed in 'bread and butter' treatment such as fillings, extractions and dentures. Nevertheless, new graduates still faced a learning curve in Britain.

The Cork dental emigrants differed from other Irish expatriates in two significant ways: they experienced little anti-Irish racism, and they frequently returned to Ireland. Oral testimony from numerous Cork graduates indicates an absence of significant anti-Irish discrimination or abuse. This likely reflected the dentists' elevated social standing, which seemed to have protected them from the very real anti-Irish sentiment at that time. Cork graduates also embraced their middle-class respectability, which emphasised integration and downplayed cultural and political differences in Britain. In this way, dentists (and other professionals, such as doctors, engineers, civil servants and engineers) separated themselves from the broader Irish migrant community in Britain, which was considerably poorer and less educated. When interacting with their fellow exiles, Irish dentists frequently preferred the respectable confines of the Irish Club or the National University of Ireland Club (both in London) rather than the boisterous dance halls of Cricklewood and Kilburn. That said, some exiles kept a foot planted firmly in both camps.

It should also be noted that many of the emigrant Cork graduates made their way back to Ireland during the ensuing years. Those who left during the 1950s could attribute their homecoming to timing, as the 1960s became a period of strong economic expansion in Ireland. However, later generations of dentists also found a return path to Ireland, often arriving home with enough money to buy their way into a practice. They brought with them exposure to the latest dental innovations and advanced ideas of practice management, which helped raise the standards of the Irish dental profession. Yet the boat journey became a one-way trip for many, even those who, like most emigrants, believed their departure to be temporary. Emigration has remained a feature of Irish dental education in the ensuing generations, as the school's more recent graduates can attest.

LEADERSHIP

The successful deanship of Israel Scher abruptly ended in the autumn of 1949. Scher had quarrelled with some members of staff when he authorised student purchases of equipment cabinets without prior approval of the staff. This escalated into a full-blown row that featured a faction of the staff demanding an apology from Scher, who ultimately resigned (staff member John O'Sullivan also

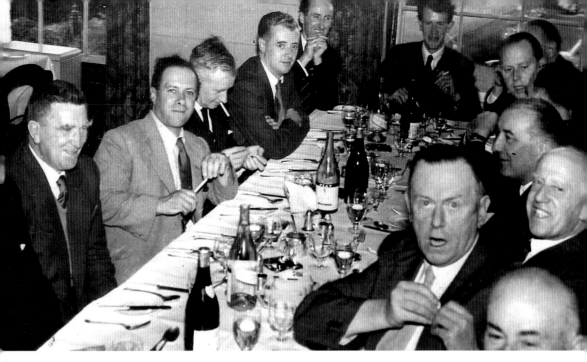

resigned in sympathy). This was only the latest in a series of angry exchanges between Scher and some members of his staff.

Jack Daunt replaced Scher as dean. Born into one of Cork's leading merchant families, Daunt had served in the hospital since 1918. Tall and confident, Daunt projected a commanding presence, and was regarded as 'the supreme dentist' in Cork. He developed an interest in prosthetic dentistry, especially in the fabrication of upper and lower dentures. Daunt became renowned for his skilful setting up of upper front teeth to give them the 'natural look', deploying what he called the 'depressed lateral' technique. He also developed an artistry using plaster of Paris to take impressions of the upper and lower jaws, which were used in the fabrication of dentures.

While Daunt possessed the aura of an academic dean, he also represented a linkage with the old apprenticeship system. Daunt possessed an LDS, but had not pursued any higher qualification or degree during his thirty years at the hospital. Though modern dental education ultimately passed him by, Daunt kept a firm hand on the tiller over the next thirteen years.

When Israel Scher left CUDSH, his place in the school was

Jack Daunt (front right, adjusting collar), Paddy O'Riordan (second left), Eric Scher (third left, holding pen), and Paddy Hackett (head of table, with cigarette) at a Irish Dental Association Munster branch dinner, circa 1950s.
Courtesy Brian O'Riordan

THE SCHERS

The Scher family should be remembered by all CUDSH graduates. Patriarch Israel 'Issa' Scher co-founded the school, and was a long-time dean. His sons Eric and Leslie provided an academic grounding to the school at a time when it was most needed. Beyond their contributions to Irish dental education, the Scher family also linked the school to the city's small Jewish community, which was vibrant for much of the twentieth century.

Israel Scher's father emigrated to Cork, and became involved in money-lending and finance. Following Israel's education at Presentation College and the Royal College of Surgeons, he opened a popular practice on Patrick's Hill. His four sons (Leslie, Eric, Gerald and Ivor) likewise attended Presentation College, and progressed to UCC. All four received their BDS, winning numerous student awards in the process.

Leslie, Eric and Ivor joined the part-time clinical-teaching staff after graduation, with the first two achieving senior positions. Eric undertook research of the geometry of dental arcades with UCC's highly regarded anatomy professor, Michael MacConaill (formerly an IRA officer during the War of Independence). The charismatic Leslie secured a Fellowship of Dental Surgery from the Royal College of Surgeons, Edinburgh. Both Eric and Leslie published multiple peer-reviewed research articles during their teaching careers.

The Schers were built similarly (short and stout), with the exception of their younger and taller brother Ivor. He enjoyed an outstanding rugby career at Presentation College, as scrum half and captain of its Munster Cup-winning side. His father forbade Ivor from playing rugby with Munster, afraid that he would ruin his hands and his dental career. He quit rugby, but for some time secretly played soccer under the name 'Ivor Smith' to escape his father's wrath. He stayed with dentistry despite receiving invitations to professional-club trials.

The Scher family mirrored the broader experience of the Dublin and Cork Jewish communities. They hailed from a rural area of Lithuania, arriving at the same time and from the same place as much of Ireland's Jewish population.

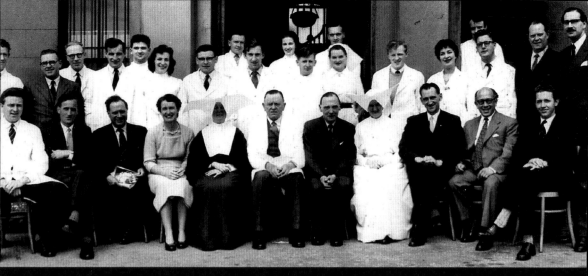

Many of their offspring found success in the professions, including dentistry. However, a demographic decline within the Jewish community accelerated in the 1950s and 1960s. With diminished marriage prospects for their children, the brothers emigrated. Ivor moved to Israel, where he renewed his friendship with classmate and fellow clinical instructor David Birkhahn (BDS 1951), another member of the Cork Jewish community (his sister Shirley also qualified; BDS 1958). Eric went into private practice in Brighton, taught at the Royal Dental Hospital in London, and became a president of the British Society of Prosthodontics. Later, he was appointed senior lecturer and consultant in prosthetics at Queen's University Belfast School of Dentistry, teaching there until his retirement in 1981. His colleagues established the Dr Eric Scher Prize, awarded to the top performer in the prosthetics segment of the final BDS exam. Leslie went into practice in England and moved away from teaching. However, the Scher dental-education legacy has been carried on by his son Dr Edwin ('Eddie') Scher. Practising in Walpole Street, London, Eddie is an internationally renowned expert in implantology, and has lectured on the subject at dental schools around the globe.

Eddie Scher's attendance at the CUDSH centenary celebration was a highlight of the event. The warm reception he received from UCC President Michael Murphy, School Dean Finbarr Allen and Cork alumni testified to the high esteem and affection the Scher name still commands within the Cork dental community.

Eric Scher (front, 3rd from left) and Leslie Scher (front, 2nd from right) with hospital staff and students, 1958: (back, left to right) D. O'Driscoll, B. O'Driscoll, L. Liddy, C. Foley; (centre, left to right) P. Hackett, R. Gamble, T. Walsh, B. Cussen, B. O'Connor, R. Devlin, L. O'Connell, T. Costelloe, B. O'Riordan, S. Downey, N. Coakley, S. Birkhahn, J. Power, J. O'Sullivan, D. Birkhahn; (front, left to right) A. McHale, P. Gleeson, E. Scher, B. Ryan, Sr Monica, J. Daunt, Prof. Roche, Matron, North Infirmary Hospital, A. Barrett, L. Scher, K. Nolan. COURTESY LIAM O'CONNELL

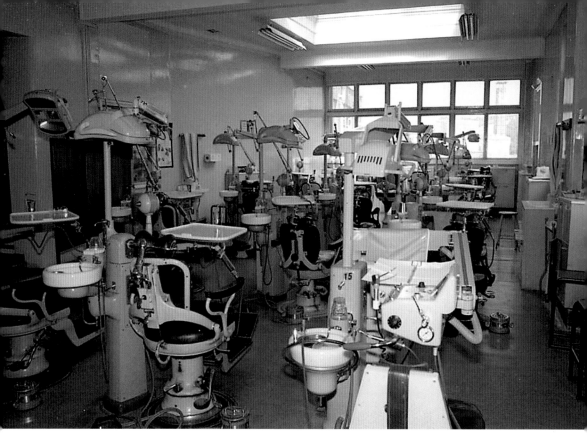

*Old dental hospital main
conservation room.*
COURTESY P.J. BYRNE

ably filled by his sons Leslie (FDS) and Eric (BDSI, M.Sc.), both strong dental educators in their own right. Each was a top graduate of the Cork University Dental School and Hospital, possessing strong scholastic and research instincts. They were among the very few staff members to publish academic articles. Academically minded students gravitated to the Scher brothers, who could be counted on to produce dental instruments from their pockets or the latest journal articles to stimulate discussion. They filled an intellectual void at the school that became more apparent as the years progressed. Jack Daunt retained supporters within the school, who appreciated his natural leadership skills.

Throughout Daunt's reign, he feuded with the Scher brothers. The relationship had gotten off to a rocky start during Eric Scher's first year on staff, when he spurned professional advice from Daunt in front of students. Daunt demanded Scher's removal from the faculty, and objected when the staff required only a written apology from Eric. Relations could only have worsened following Daunt's controversial replacement of Israel Scher. The staff-meeting minutes from the period record numerous disagreements between the two factions, often initiated by Daunt. Some observers detected anti-Semitism from Daunt, while others attributed the bad blood solely to professional rivalry. Both Schers possessed superior academic qualifications to Daunt, and Leslie emerged as a competitor for the deanship in later years. As a result, inter-staff relations remained testy throughout the 1950s. Unfortunately, similar acrimony reappeared within CUDSH periodically in the following decades.

THE 1961 VISITATION

The 1950s were a woeful time for Irish higher education, with university facilities antiquated, undersized and often lacking in essential teaching equipment. Full-time staff were perceived to be a luxury rather than a necessity, as evidenced by the absence of full-time staff in UCC's law and engineering faculties until the 1970s. The lack of full-time staff in the School of Medicine resulted in scathing visitation reports that threatened its accreditation. Indeed, in the late 1950s a number of states in the United States did not recognise the UCC medical degree.

In dentistry, as in other higher-education sectors, Ireland had not kept up with European norms. Since the Second World War, British dental education had progressed swiftly, as hospitals improved their facilities and hired full-time teachers. By 1961 no British dental school had less than fifteen full-time teaching staff (either college lecturers or hospital clinical instructors), while the Cork and Dublin schools possessed none. Both Irish dental schools were housed in creaking hospitals that even their most devoted defenders would regard as lacking.

Recognising the challenges presented by the new National

Health Service, British medical authorities launched the Teviot Interdepartmental Committee. Its 1944 *Teviot Report* called for a standardisation of dental education, including more rigorous screening of dental schools whose graduates were allowed to practise in Britain. Ultimately, the British General Dental Council established visitation committees to inspect accredited dental schools so as to maintain minimum teaching standards.

CUDSH authorities recognised that their school had fallen behind those in the UK. In 1955 a special staff meeting considered the shortcomings of Cork's BDS course, which was six months shorter than British degree programmes. That same year, the CUDSH lobbied the North Infirmary governing body to hire full-time staff, warning that without such an appointment it faced closure as a teaching hospital. Ultimately, the North Infirmary and university funded two half-time teaching positions with an annual salary of £600 each, which were filled in mid-1957 by Eric Scher and Barry Collins. CUDSH also began to pay teaching staff on a sessional basis, though members received a paltry £2.20 per two-hour teaching session. There was an internal attempt to replace Dean Jack Daunt with Leslie Scher, who was better positioned to place the school on an academic trajectory. However, Daunt defeated Scher on a narrow eleven-to-seven vote.

Nationally, Irish dental educators scrambled to improve teaching standards prior to pending inspections from the British Dental Council. In mid-1957 a special committee was formed to 'safeguard reciprocity of degrees'; it was comprised of the minister for education, Cork and Dublin dental-hospital authorities, dental officers in Cork and Dublin, and the deans of the UCD, UCC, TCD and Royal College of Surgeons in Ireland dental schools. Yet little state investment in dental education was forthcoming.

Aware of their tenuous position, CUDSH staff members tried to make last-minute improvements. They hired architect J.R. Boyd Barrett to draw up plans to expand the hospital, but could not raise enough funds to begin construction (Catholic Bishop Cornelius Lucey assisted their fund-raising). The staff also created a new student recording system and they restructured teaching departments. However, in some ways their efforts resembled a rearrangement of deck chairs on the *Titanic*. In 1958 the hospital staff again appealed to UCC for more space, improved accommodations and full-time paid staff, which they considered 'essential to bring our schools to a level comparable with others'. The British General Dental Council Visitation Committee (responsible for recognising dental degrees in the UK) would make similar demands, albeit with considerable more force behind them.

The 1961 Cork visitation committee featured leading medical educators from Britain: Sir Harry Platt (former president, Royal College of Surgeons), Kenneth P. Liddelow (professor of prosthetic dentistry, King's College Hospital Dental School, London), John Boyes (professor of dental surgery, Royal College of Surgeons of Edinburgh) and Professor G.H. Bell (professor of physiology, University College Dundee). Like all examinations, the visitation created excitement and nervousness at CUDSH, as each department readied itself for inspection on 1–2 May 1961. Staff anticipated a negative report. The only question was the extent of the damage.

The visitation-committee's report offers a fascinating snapshot of the school's state in 1961. The inspectors recognised dedicated (if underqualified) teachers, though they found obvious fault with the absence of full-time staff. CUDSH's professionalism and standard of care were judged to be satisfactory, while suggestions were made to better integrate course instruction with clinical work. Yet the committee could not ignore the appalling condition of the dental hospital itself. An extended quotation provides a glimpse of the primitive facilities:

> The dental department is housed in one floor in an old
> building with facilities which are totally inadequate for

teaching dental surgery up to the standards required at the present day. There is no proper waiting accommodation for the patients and a draughty balcony is used. A small, ill-equipped room is used for the examination of all out-patients and for the local anaesthesia and for periodontal treatment. Sterilisation facilities are minimal. The main clinic, which is equipped with twelve chairs, is used for all clinical instruction and treatment, except prosthetics; the equipment is old-fashioned and much worn and only two proper dental units are installed. There are no small demonstration or treatment surgeries, no photographic or X-ray department, and no rooms or facilities for the staff whatsoever. Library facilities are poor.

Representatives of University College Cork, the North Infirmary and CUDSH expressed their willingness to make the desired changes. Accepting their word, the committee spared CUDSH's accreditation, or, more precisely, stayed its execution for four years. It delivered two conditions: appoint full-time staff and construct a new dental hospital. The report warned:

> We think that the present teaching and facilities at Cork compared with those at the other schools we have visited are barely sufficient and that each year that passes without change will make them less so.

CUDSH was given until 1965 to get its house in order. The Dublin dental hospital also received an 'insufficient' rating, and was granted a similar four-year reprieve.

MODERNISATION

Like an old car shifting gears, CUDSH slowly made adjustments, and then accelerated with an uncomfortable bump.

Reading the writing on the wall, Leslie Scher left Cork for England at the end of 1961, following his brother Eric, who in 1959 had taken up a teaching position at the Royal Dental Hospital in London. Their departure severed the Scher family's forty-eight-year relationship with the school. They should be remembered as the most influential figures during the school's first half-century.

Jack Daunt also stepped down, though his resignation took effect after the dust settled in 1963. At that time, the National University of Ireland conferred Daunt with an honorary doctorate, LL D. His replacement, Barry Collins (BDS 1938), became the school's first dean who was also an alumnus. Born in Cork, Collins enjoyed a lively career in the Royal Navy during the Second World War. He had been posted to HMS *Hood* but was not on-board when she was sunk by the German battleship *Bismark*, taking all but three of the crew with her. He then became dental officer aboard the cruiser HMS *Birmingham*, and saw active service across African and Mediterranean waters. When he eventually returned to Cork, he set up a successful practice on Patrick's Hill, and became president of the Irish Dental Association in 1958. A popular teacher of conservative dentistry since joining the staff in 1949, he was a warm man with a good sense of humour. Collins was also remembered for his skilled precision, which included demonstrating to students a chiselling technique to prepare cavities without a drill. Though he led the school for only two years, he provided a safe pair of hands during the crucial transition period. School historian Ray Gamble would later recall: 'Barry Collins, he was the man that kept the school together.'

By 1963, a year following the publication of the damaging visitation report, little movement was perceived by the school staff, especially on the relatively straightforward question of hiring full-time staff. The staff had recommended the appointment of one full-time hospital director, and three full-time hospital-department heads. They had also notified university authorities that in 1961, without accounting for salaries, the hospital operated on the shoestring budget of £2,500. In 1962 the total payments to the school's ten part-time teaching staff came to just £900 annually. In their opinion, hospital spending resulted from 'economy which is not in keeping with a reasonable standard of dental treatment'. Despite the urgency, dental-school staff believed the hospital and university authorities had taken few of the steps required to bring CUDSH up to standard prior to the critical 1965 visitation.

Upping the ante in July of 1963, the dental-school staff submitted a letter to the North Infirmary Committee of Management that read in part:

Ger Fitzgerald BDS conferring, 1955.

Unless full-time positions are established within a reasonable time, it would be morally wrong to continue to accept

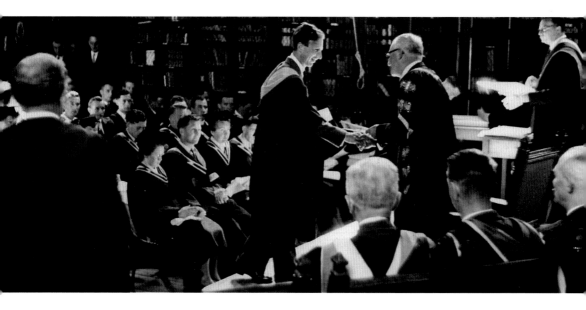

students under conditions that prevail at present. They feel, therefore, that unless a full-time director is appointed immediately and the further full-time positions are filled within the next six months, it would be preferable to dissolve the school.

The protest spurred into action UCC President Dr H. St John Atkins. Speaking at a summer conferring a couple of weeks later, Atkins expressed surprise that the dental-school staff had first approached the North Infirmary and not the university, and assured his audience that the dental hospital would remain open. Though Atkins had neglected to mention UCC's repeated deafness to numerous earlier appeals from the dental-school staff, he had at last publicly committed the university to maintaining dental education.

The following month, a committee was formed to save the school, comprised of Norman Butler (dental-school staff) and university officials including President Atkins. A meeting was arranged with the relevant government ministers, Seán MacEntee

BDS class of 1963, as first-year dental students in 1959: (back, left to right) R. Donegan, F. Daly, J. Rafferty, K. Quinlan, B. O'Callaghan; (centre, left to right) G. Cuddigan, I. Rosenberg, J. Walsh, T. Holland; (front, left to right) C. O'Brien, A. Jordan, F. Quane, J. O'Connor. Courtesy Frank Daly

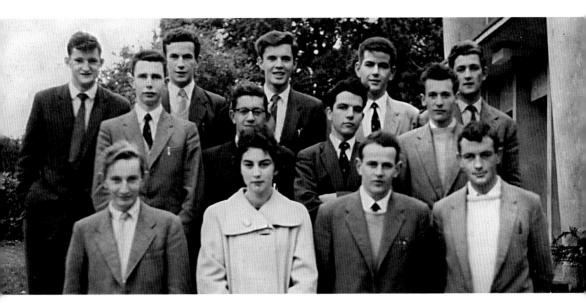

(minister for health) and Dr Patrick Hillery (minister for education). Norman Butler and Gordon Russell represented CUDSH, while the dean of the medical faculty, Dr Paddy Kiely, acted for UCC. The intervention proved highly satisfactory. Ultimately the government agreed to:

(a)   Build a new dental hospital in Cork (to be attached to the proposed Regional Hospital at Wilton, Cork);
(a)   Finance four full-time chairs in dentistry at UCC, one of whom was to be the CUDSH director of dental studies;
(a)   Provide an immediate capital grant of £17,000 (later increased to £30,000) to update antiquated equipment.

APPOINTMENTS

The university moved forward with its appointment of four full-time faculty members. Chairs were established in dental surgery, conservation, prosthetics and orthodontics. Appointments were made in June 1964, though only three of the four chairs were filled. The new full-time dental professors were J. Gordon Russell (chair of dental surgery), Brian Barrett (chair of conservative dentistry) and Mary Hegarty (chair of orthodontics).

Mary Hegarty (BDS 1955) became the first female dental professor in Ireland, and enjoyed popularity with students during her forty-year service to the school. The next appointment of a woman came in the 1990s, which was indicative of Irish higher-education's glacial pace towards gender equality. The second appointee, Gordon Russell, had secured both a Fellowship in Dental Surgery from the Royal College of Surgeons of England (FDSRCSE) and a Fellowship Faculty of Dentistry, Royal College of Surgeons in Ireland (FFDRCSI). He was also doubly qualified, having obtained an MB in addition to a BDS. He took over the deanship from Barry Collins, though by this point the title became

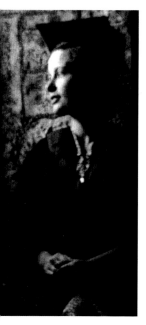

Professor Mary Hegarty at her 1955 BDS conferring.

honorary rather than administrative. The school's prosthetics chair remained unfilled until Dr William McCullough's hiring in 1969. An internationally recognised researcher, McCullough built up a solid prosthetics department while undertaking advanced work in dental materials.

The other full-time appointment, Brian Barrett, became arguably the most important figure in the history of the Cork dental school. Tall and charismatic, Professor Barrett filled a leadership vacuum within the dental school. Like Gordon Russell, he possessed an MB, BDS, FDSRCSE and FFDRCSI. During his twenty-five-year reign as director of dental studies (which assumed the responsibilities of school dean), Barrett proved himself an able administrator and first-rate advocate for the school. When the school faced a new crisis in the 1970s, Barrett led the institution's tenacious defence.

RESEARCH & FACILITIES

Using the government's capital grant and additional support from UCC, the hospital underwent an upgrade. New equipment included an X-ray machine (housed in a specially constructed X-ray department) and an autoclave to sterilise instruments. The hospital interior was reconfigured, adding space and a second entrance. Air-rotor drills also came into the hospital for the first time, which dramatically reduced cavity preparation time.

New premises were secured in Moylan's Lane (used as a prosthetics laboratory) and at a converted residential home at 4 St John's Terrace. The latter became the school's research centre. Much of the innovation was driven by the Health (Fluoridation of Water Supplies) Act of 1960, which empowered the Department of Health to fluoridate water supplies. The Act included a monitoring provision intended to detect dental-decay levels on a regular and ongoing basis so as to judge the effectiveness of fluoridation. In 1965 the Department of Health established a unit in Cork dental school – called 'Special Studies in Dental Caries and Fluorides' – to carry out the monitoring function. Cork graduate Dr Chris Collins headed the unit, which was linked to CUDSH's new Department of Preventive and Paediatric Dentistry and housed at 4 St John's Terrace. The special unit was replaced by the Oral Health Services Research Centre in 1983.

The special unit carried out a number of landmark studies on fluoride use in Ireland. A 1969 survey randomly sampled four-to-eleven-year-old Cork city schoolchildren, who had been consuming fluoridated water since 1965. The Cork city study results showed that their decay levels were substantially lower than those recorded in pre-fluoridated baseline studies of the same age group. The special unit also investigated alternative methods for introducing fluoride where water fluoridation was not feasible. The 1970 Fermoy (County Cork) Mouth Rinse Study randomly assigned participating children to study and control groups. Children in the study group rinsed with a sodium-fluoride solution, while children in the control group rinsed with distilled water. Supervised rinsing was conducted fortnightly in the schools. The final report demonstrated that the study group experienced a highly significant reduction in the incidence of dental caries compared with the control group. Beyond its important fluoridation work, the special unit entered new areas of dental research during the ensuing years.

STATE DENTAL SERVICE

CUDSH in this period benefitted from an expansion of the state dental service, which provided jobs for recent graduates, research opportunities, and wider public appreciation of dental treatment. Cork graduates treated public patients around the country, often in primitive conditions. Gerald Fitzgerald recalled visiting locales in County Dublin without electricity or running water. Often, he worked with a bucket of water and furiously pedalled his treadle machine, which required forty-five minutes' drilling to prepare a cavity for filling. While undertaking clinic work in remote County Kerry schools during winter, Willie Palmer remembered starting his day by chiselling ice from windows and his water bucket. The high level of tooth extractions in these clinics cannot be overstated. What might be called the 'sixty rule' reflects the state of affairs: in 1960 sixty per cent of Cork city adults over the age of sixty had no natural teeth.

The growth of the public-health dentistry sector can be seen in the careers of the CUDSH class of 1955, whose graduates included Colm Bell, principal dental officer with the Southern Health Board; Gerald Fitzgerald, principal dental officer in the Eastern Health Board; Frank Gilligan, senior clinical dental surgeon with the Southern Health Board; and Frank McGrath, senior clinical dental officer with the Southern Health Board. Many public-sector dentists felt a sense of vocation to provide critical services to their community.

Denis O'Mullane's experience with the Cork Dental Authority in 1965 illustrates the challenges facing public-sector dentists during Ireland's modernisation in the 1960s. As a dental surgeon focused mainly on emergency extractions, O'Mullane visited three dental clinics on a rotational basis: Clonakilty (in the town hall), Skibbereen (in the county-council offices) and Dunmanway. He subsequently took on clinics in Bantry (Bantry Hospital), Castletownbere (county-council offices) and Schull (Schull Cottage Hospital). At Dunmanway, the clinic was situated in a room off the Laurel Bar, owned by Mr and Mrs Paddy O'Regan. Their son Barry O'Regan (BDS 1983, FDS, MB, BCH, BAO) is now employed as an oral and maxillofacial surgeon in Scotland, while their daughter, Colette O'Regan (BDS 1978), also qualified.

Dentistry increasingly became accessible to all segments of Irish society, as public-sector dentists pushed into the most remote

TOM 'BOSS' WALSH:
DENTAL MECHANIC

In the first half-century of the Cork dental school, the
BDS programme heavily emphasised the teaching of dental
mechanics. Students learned various mechanical skills,
including preparing metal for crowns, creating filling material,
and constructing dentures. As such, students often depended on
the kindness of the hospital dental technician. Perhaps the most
colourful of these was Tom 'Boss' Walsh.

Boss Walsh was born in Cork in 1911, and educated at the
North Monastery Secondary School. He became an apprentice
dental mechanic in 1926, and found a job in Andy O'Mahony's
dental practice in Winthrop Street, Cork. For a number of
years, Walsh worked as a dental mechanic in the morning, and
then in the afternoon and evening was employed as an usher at
the Savoy Cinema on Patrick Street. That job introduced Walsh
to his future wife, Monica Harty, who worked in the Savoy as a
cashier.

In the 1940s Walsh joined the practice of Joe Ollivere, who
was closely associated with the dental school. During 1948, with
Ollivere's support Boss Walsh secured the position of dental
curator at the dental hospital. Already a capable craftsman,
Walsh proved a natural teacher. Students appreciated his
patience, good humour and willingness to offer extra time
when it was needed. His large personality ensured the personal
popularity of Boss Walsh within the hospital. He especially liked
to regale students with tall tales of his daring do, some of which
were true.

Outside the hospital, Walsh enjoyed an active life within Cork city. He remained engaged with both the Fianna Fáil and Clan na Poblachta political parties. Walsh also devoted himself to the St Vincent de Paul Society and the Prisoners' Aid Group, which helped released prisoners find work. But Boss Walsh was best known for his devotion to music. He was a leading member of the Cork Grand Opera Group, which staged operas at the Coliseum Theatre and Cork Opera House during the 1950s. Boss Walsh also performed with the Cork City Choral Society. He joined the group's successful tour of the 1958 World's Fair in Brussels, where it offered traditional Irish songs and dancing. The Belgium touring party contained a strong dental-school influence, including Boss Walsh and dental students Denis O'Mullane and Seán McCarthy. The group's deputy conductor, Rita Mulcahy, was married to Cork graduate and part-time lecturer Pat Gleeson.

Tom 'Boss' Walsh.
COURTESY TOM WALSH

Boss Walsh relished his time at the Cork dental hospital, and closely followed the careers of his former students. He took great pride in their achievements. University College Cork formally recognised his devotion to the institution in 1977, when it awarded him an honorary master's degree in science. He died two years later, and will be remembered in the dental school as one of its great characters.

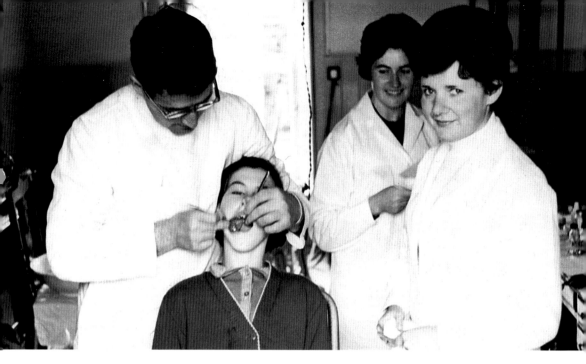

Denis O'Mullane
with dental nurses
Margaret Lee (back) and
Joyce Daly (front), treating
a Cape Clear islander in
Cotter's pub, 1966.
COURTESY DENIS O'MULLANE

parts of Ireland. The dental expedition to Cape Clear Island offers a case study of this effort. In 1966 the Cork Health Authority's chief dental officer, George MacSweeney, authorised dental treatment for the Cape Clear islanders. A temporary clinic would be opened on the island by Cork Health Authority staff, namely dental surgeons Vincent Bluett and Denis O'Mullane (both Cork graduates) and dental nurses Joyce Daly and Margaret Lee.

The team brought with them two dental chairs, air rotors, air compressors, sterilisers, and surgical and restorative equipment, which were transported by a fishing trawler operated by Kieran Cotter. Since Cotter also owned a pub near the main pier on Cape Clear Island, the clinic was set up in the pub's snug. The remarkable Cotter was also an engineer (a UCC graduate) running his own electrical generator, which was the island's sole source of power at that time. Fortunately, dental surgeon Vincent Bluett (BDS 1957) was both an accomplished electrician and an accomplished dentist, thus ensuring a smooth collaboration.

On 13 September 1966, the team began treating patients in two operating chairs. Extractions and fillings were provided for adult medical-card holders and approximately fifty schoolchildren. At the end of the two weeks, many islanders had received their first ever comprehensive treatment.

Throughout these years, inspired public-sector dentists made similar inroads across Ireland. To ordinary Irish citizens, dentistry had become part of basic health-care requirements, and was no longer a synonym for tooth removal.

EXPANSION

As Ireland modernised during the 1960s, state investment in higher education increased. Universities constructed new buildings, created college chairs and added degree programmes. Scholarships and other financial-aid schemes made universities accessible to a new generation of Irish people. The introduction of free secondary education further expanded the third-level student population.

In Cork, dental postgraduate degrees became more common in the 1960s. The school's first recognised postgraduate course had taken place during 1948. In the early 1960s Norman Butler and Chris Collins secured Master of Dental Surgery (MDS) degrees, while Joe Ollivere achieved a Higher Dental Degree (HDD). Denis O'Mullane became the school's first dental Ph.D. in 1971, the first such degree awarded to a dentist in Ireland. The addition of postgraduate degree courses during these years frequently complemented the research undertaken by the special unit at 4 St John's Terrace.

At this time, UCC also became more directly involved in hospital operations, as university bursar Jim Hurley (a much storied GAA figure and War of Independence flying-column leader) added the school to his administrative responsibilities. The North Infirmary began to disengage from administering the dental hospital, a process that concluded in 1968. Thereafter, UCC took over governance of the hospital, which it was agreed would be on a temporary basis. However, the structure has not changed

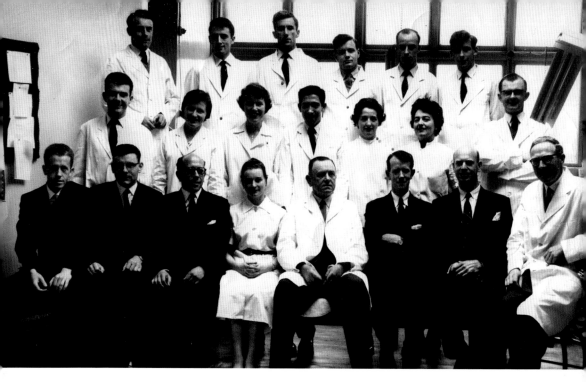

BDS class, 1960:
(back, left to right) C. Foley,
D. O'Mullane, L. Shalloe,
S. O'Luasa, J. O'Donoghue,
B. O'Gorman;
(centre, left to right)
S. McCarthy, B. O'Sullivan,
K. Moloney, M. Nunan,
S. Gould, N. Kaminska,
D. Magauran;
(front, left to right)
D. Crofts, L. O'Connell,
L. Scher, S. Downey,
J. Daunt, P. Hackett,
G. Russell, T. Walsh.
Courtesy Denis O'Mullane

in the ensuing forty-five years, much to the discomfort of UCC authorities.

In 1965 the school received a second visit from the General Dental Council. The visitation committee found improvements in curriculum, course syllabi and the final dental examination. Hospital facilities were still deemed inadequate, but school authorities assured the examiners that a new dental hospital would soon be erected alongside the pending Regional Hospital at Wilton. The visitation committee decided to continue to recognise the Cork degree.

Like the rest of Ireland during the 1960s, the Cork University Dental School and Hospital had adapted to a rapidly changing society. The school altered its course and seemed to be sailing into calm seas. Construction of a new dental hospital would soon begin, and its completion would bring the institution long-term security. Unfortunately, the new hospital proved much more difficult to build than anticipated. Within a few short years, CUDSH officials once again embarked on a bitter struggle to save the school. Their victory would take nine gruelling years.

4

BUILDING A NEW HOSPITAL & SAVING THE SCHOOL

THE Cork University Dental School and Hospital began the 1960s in precarious health, but made a steady recovery throughout the decade. By 1970 CUDSH had improved its teaching, curriculum and overall quality of instruction. Yet the decrepit and deteriorating dental-hospital structure threatened the school's future existence.

Having demanded a new hospital in 1961 and again in 1965, the General Dental Council Visitation Committee in 1969 expressed exasperation at the lack of progress:

> It is obvious to us that, without a new building, the Cork Dental School cannot survive as a viable entity … Ingenuity and contrivance have made the totally inadequate accommodation of the building just about viable as a dental hospital and school …

In 1963 the government had promised to build a dental complex alongside the new Regional General Hospital (now called Cork University Hospital) at Wilton, Cork. Yet delivering that new dental hospital turned out to be much more difficult than expected. At times, observers reduced the issue to a new round in the long-standing rivalry between Cork and Dublin, dismissing Cork objections as 'Leeside begrudgery'. Yet in doing so they ignored a fundamental question about Irish dental health and education: would the state be best served by one or two dental schools? From a Cork perspective, a satisfactory answer was delivered by a broad coalition of CUDSH advocates, who engaged in nine years of protracted struggle.

KAIM-CAUDLE, THE HEA REPORT & UNIVERSITY RATIONALISATION

The conflict began in 1969 with the publication of the Economic and Social Research Institute study *Dental Services in Ireland*. Written by the economics professor Peter Kaim-Caudle, the report recommended a single, large dental school in Ireland rather than two medium-sized institutions in Dublin and Cork. Critics of the 'Kaim-Caudle report' (as it became known) objected to the author's lack of public-health and dental expertise. Profound changes to dental education had been recommended on financial grounds by an economist unfamiliar with dentistry. Despite these shortcomings, the Kaim-Caudle report quickly found prominent backers within the National University of Ireland, then busily reorganising Irish higher education.

Rationalisation in Irish universities had become a national priority in the late 1960s. The NUI's flagship effort was the ill-fated proposed merger between Trinity College Dublin and University College Dublin. Extensive negotiations over TCD's status were part of a broader third-level restructuring, which included consolidations and eliminations of duplicate programmes and faculties. After private discussions between top university officials, the government released a series of recommendations in April 1970.

Numerous disciplines were affected by the NUI plan, including medicine, science, law, agriculture, commerce, veterinary medicine, pharmacy and engineering. UCC would retain its medical, agriculture and law schools, and was offered an expensive new computer-science department. However, citing budget reasons, the report also suggested closing the Cork University Dental School and Hospital. TCD would then serve as the state's sole dental educator.

Some academics were troubled by NUI decisions that lacked transparency and appeared arbitrary. Faculties lowered onto the chopping block fumed at the lack of prior consultation, denying them an opportunity to justify their existence. At the convocation of the NUI a month after the report's release, one such head of school protested publicly. Dean Patrick McGeady, of the imperilled UCD veterinary school, thundered:

> It is a sorry day for university education in Ireland when these universities disregard what is required to produce the best graduate in a particular faculty, but instead by a process of bargaining, like tinkers at a fair, decide UCD will take faculty A, TCD will take faculty B, and in faculty C they split the difference and take a piece of each, with possibly some smaller faculty thrown in here and there as luck's penny.

Replying on behalf of the NUI, the noted TCD geneticist Professor George Dawson defended the rationalisation of third-level faculties around the country. He justified the closure of the Cork dental school on both economic and educational grounds, insinuating that Cork did not stand 'a good chance of being a good school'. He added: 'In the long term it is difficult to imagine a dental school in Cork doing other than struggling to keep up with the standards of the Dublin school.'

UCC director of dental studies, Brian Barrett, promptly answered Dawson in a letter that appeared in national newspapers. Barrett clarified that the NUI justified closing CUDSH on financial rather than educational grounds. He further argued that Dawson's 'gravely damaging' suggestion of Cork's academic inferiority to Dublin was Dawson's alone, and had 'the added disadvantage of being untrue'. Dawson subsequently suggested that Barrett had misconstrued his remarks, which he meant to refer to CUDSH's future prospects rather than its current standards. Such a fine distinction may have been lost on Dawson's audience.

Facing an existential threat, the dental school mobilised

community support in Cork. Protests against the proposed closure promptly came from the North Infirmary governing body, Cork Health Authority, Cork Corporation and the Munster branch of the Irish Dental Association. Noel Walsh, who would emerge as a key leader within CUDSH, entered the fray for the first time as president of the Irish Dental Students' Association. He denounced the denial of 'dental education to all except residents of Dublin', and was first to float the idea of a public petition to save the school.

Initially, UCC authorities proved less than helpful. During the NUI rationalisation negotiations, Professor Patrick Quinlan represented UCC on the joint committee that prepared specific recommendations. His status as UCC's chair of mathematical physics contributed to the perception that the university had swapped dentistry for a new computer-science faculty, since the latter was of special interest to Quinlan. (To add insult to injury, Professor Quinlan subsequently became a national spokesman against water fluoridation. Dentistry later shared close quarters with the Computer Science Department on the UCC campus, in the so-called 'Sky-Lab' atop the Kane Building.) UCC President McCarthy had also participated in high-level NUI–TCD nego-tiations and had agreed with its recommendations. His academic background further weighed against the dental school, as he had previously served as a statistician at the Economic and Social Research Institute, the publisher of the Kaim-Caudle report. Dental-school advocates felt McCarthy did not truly agree with their arguments to retain dentistry. In the critical weeks after the release of the NUI proposals, McCarthy offered only tepid support for the dental school, noting the length of time before rationalisation came into effect and the financial burden CUDSH placed on the university budget. The UCC School of Medicine also remained largely silent on the controversy, which added to the dental-school's bunker mentality.

Fortunately, dentistry found reliable friends within the UCC faculty. The UCC Academic Staff Association quickly passed a motion calling on the UCC governing body to safeguard the dental school. Critical support followed from the governing body, which unanimously opposed the loss of dentistry. This pressured President McCarthy to take up the mantle of protector of the dental school, albeit belatedly. Though nothing was planned for the moment, CUDSH authorities readied themselves for a fight by marshalling data and arguments against closure.

Additional alarms sounded when Taoiseach Jack Lynch visited the dental hospital a year later, in March 1971. After praising water-fluoridation research undertaken in Cork, Lynch addressed the future of the dental school. He recognised the school's contribution to Munster's public health, and acknowledged the need for a new dental hospital. However, the Taoiseach also emphasised the high cost of dental education, tying the question to limited national resources and broader strategic goals for higher education. Ultimately, Lynch did little to reassure an anxious institution located in his own parliamentary constituency.

At the end of 1971, the Cork Hospitals Board prepared to invite tenders for the construction of the new general hospital and dental hospital at Wilton. Simultaneously, the Department of Education readied the release of its *Report on University Reorganisation* completed by the Higher Education Authority (HEA). A key recommendation of the HEA report was closure of CUDSH. With this finding in mind, the Department of Education asked the Cork Hospitals Board in January 1972 to omit the dental hospital from its pending construction plans. This would prevent a fait accompli, whereby the cost of a newly built dental hospital would compel the department to keep the dental school open. The compliant Cork Hospitals Board dropped all references to the dental hospital in the tender documentation. Bids would be accepted for the construction of the general hospital only. This decoupling of the two construction projects increased the likelihood that the new dental-hospital initiative would be abandoned.

The situation worsened with the release of the long-awaited HEA's *Report on University Reorganisation* in July 1972. If implemented, TCD would host the state's single dental school, with UCD and the Royal College of Surgeons receiving considerations in other areas.

The HEA report had been commissioned to facilitate ambitious restructuring of university education in the Dublin area. A primary goal had been the consolidation of the multiple medical schools in Dublin (operated by TCD, UCD and the Royal College of Surgeons). However, the HEA report failed to integrate the Dublin medical schools into a single unit, explaining how 'in view of the extremely complicated Universities-cum-Hospital problems and the profoundly emotional issues involved in medical education it would be unwise to press the matter further'. Brian Barrett unfavourably compared the HEA report's dental decision with its unwillingness to rationalise Dublin's medical-education facilities. He wrote: 'when it came to removing an education facility and health service from Cork and placing it 160 miles away in Dublin, it would appear that no issues, emotional or otherwise, stood in its way'. His Leeside perspective was echoed by Mary Leland in an *Irish Times* opinion piece written at the beginning of the controversy: 'Rationalisation is what happens to Cork; regionalisation is what never seems to be proposed for the Dublin universities'. It should also be noted that advocates of a single dental school always assumed that the single national institution would be located in Dublin rather than Cork. They never justified that preference, nor felt that it required explanation, which further fuelled feelings of injustice in Cork.

BRIAN BARRETT:
ACADEMIC, ADMINISTRATOR & LEADER

Professor Brian Barrett was the victorious general during the battle to save the Cork University Dental School and Hospital. His thirty-one-year service to the institution has also made him arguably the most important figure in its history.

Barrett was born in 1930 to an Irish father (a Corkman) and a South African mother residing in London. His father was a GP who served in the Royal Army Medical Corps during the First World War, and who went into private practice afterwards. The family lived on Wimpole Street, which faced German bombs during the Blitz. For his safety, Brian was evacuated to family relations in Cork city for the duration of the war. He was educated first at Presentation College and later at Clongowes Wood.

After secondary school, Brian stayed on in Ireland. He studied medicine at TCD, receiving his MB BCh in 1955, but then moved into dentistry and took a BDS (also awarded by TCD) in 1958. A gifted student, he was subsequently awarded an FDSRCSE and an FFDRCSI. At this time, he began lecturing part-time at University College Hospital, London, before securing a dental-surgery lectureship at the University of Birmingham in 1962.

Brian was one of the school's initial full-time chairs, appointed professor of conservative dentistry by UCC in 1964. He took over the school leadership from Barry Collins, assuming the title of director of dental studies, a position he held until 1991. During

Brian Barrett.

Professor Barrett's tenure, the school underwent steady improvement. Tall and slim, he was an excellent frontman for the institution. He cultivated advocates for the school, and sought colleagues committed to making Cork a centre of academic excellence. Behind the scenes, he was a top-class administrator who kept operations on an even keel, despite an often-challenging environment. Barrett remained cool and collected throughout the 'nine-years war' for the school's existence. In that regard, it is difficult to envision a better-timed appointment than his.

Professor Barrett received recognition beyond the Cork dental school. He was appointed a member of the General Dental Council (UK), served a term as president of the European Community Dental Practitioners' Advisory Committee, and was dean of the Faculty of Dentistry at the Royal College of Surgeons in Ireland. From 1979 to 1984 he was dean of the UCC School of Medicine, the only dentist to receive this distinction. He also acted as an external examiner to the University of Manchester, University of Birmingham and University of Leeds. One of his last positions was as visiting professor at the distinguished University of Witwatersrand, South Africa. Within Irish dentistry, Brian became a popular after-dinner speaker, well stocked with droll anecdotes.

Brian Barrett's tenure at Cork University Dental School and Hospital coincided with the worst crisis in the school's history. Yet he rose to the challenge with the same skill and seeming ease that he displayed when riding his motorcycle or climbing in the Pyrenees. Beneath his elegant exterior lay steely resolve, the presence of which the CUDSH community should be grateful for.

THE 'SAVE THE SCHOOL' CAMPAIGN

If President McCarthy initially seemed amenable to losing the dental school, he reversed course after receiving orders from the UCC governing body. McCarthy promptly established an ad hoc working party to challenge the HEA findings. Its members were Brian Barrett and Finbarr Corkery (of the dental school), the new UCC finance officer, Michael Kelleher, and Cork businessman F.L. Jacob, who was a member of the UCC governing body. The ad hoc group sought to challenge the arguments used to justify the school's closure. To Michael Kelleher, the HEA report's vulnerable buttress was its vague cost breakdown for educating a single dental student. This ambiguity undermined the report's critical financial conclusions. Ultimately, the ad hoc committee made a number of arguments against the HEA report, including the following:

- The proposed rationalisation did not decrease the overall number of dental students educated in the state. This meant the staff-to-student ratio (the main cost calculation) did not improve, which raised questions as to whether amalgamation would actually produce savings.
- The report's costing assumptions for a new large dental hospital in Dublin were speculative, since a site there had not yet been chosen. CUDSH, on the other hand, had already purchased a site and planned a structure, making its new-hospital costing more reliable.
- The report entirely ignored the community public-health impact of the move. This area offered the most persuasive case for retention in the ensuing public campaign.

The UCC working party detailed its objections in a counter report UCC published in early 1973. A press conference and public meeting marked the release of the working-party document, which was widely disseminated to mobilise opposition to the school's closure. President McCarthy endorsed its findings, as did the UCC governing body and Academic Council. Meanwhile, Brian Barrett sought further assistance in persuading the Department of Education to reverse the HEA findings.

Irish universities in Dublin have traditionally enjoyed easier access to influential government officials than schools located outside the capital. Yet in the early 1970s, UCC benefited from a uniquely friendly political landscape where a number of Cork city politicians held high national office. The most obvious was Taoiseach Jack Lynch, whose constituency included the dental hospital. During the 'save the school' campaign, a number of students and staff approached Lynch at various locales in the city. Lynch found himself politely listening to impassioned dental-school defensives on the Grand Parade, in the Imperial Hotel bar and in the Muskerry Golf Club, though it is unclear if these interventions affected his government's higher-education policy. Perhaps a better friend of the dental school was the less prominent Cork Fianna Fáil politician, Gus Healy TD. Disabled by a childhood accident that left him under five feet tall, Healy attributed his political success to Fr Seamus O'Flynn's inner-city youth Shakespeare theatre, The Loft, which was located very close to the dental hospital. Healy also ran a dental-mechanic laboratory, embedding him firmly within the city's dental establishment. Frequently acting behind the scenes, Healy helped the 'save the school' campaign navigate treacherous political shoals. He also served as a public advocate, raising the issue numerous times in Dáil Éireann. Sitting across from Healy was another Cork city TD, Peter Barry, a power within Fine Gael during the 1970s and 1980s. As minister for education, he forcefully intervened on the school's behalf in 1976.

Loyal school alumni quickly rallied to the standard. Remarkable support came from local dentists, acting through the Munster branch of the Irish Dental Association. Members formed a

Dental Hospital Retention Committee under the leadership of Tim Riordan (other members included Dominic Crofts, Finbarr O'Sullivan, Liam O'Connell, Tony Canty, Louis Buckley and Patrick O'Connor.) Passing the hat, the Retention Committee raised a significant fighting fund with which it hired Dermot Breen's public-relations firm. Influential in Irish cinema, Breen founded the Cork Film Festival and served as its director from 1956 to 1978, and was the Irish film censor from 1972 to 1978. Breen subsequently waged a clever marketing campaign on behalf of the Cork dental school, organising events, contacting politicians and placing favourable press stories.

At the end of the year, the school unleashed its secret weapon: the dental students. During a time of national and international youth political activism, Cork students needed little prodding to take to the streets. The initial agitation took the form of a one-day student strike that shut the dental hospital. Tom Boland (BDS 1974) led the entire student body (eighty-six students) onto Patrick Street, where they distributed four thousand leaflets calling for the construction of a new hospital. The strike action was taken in conjunction with Dublin dental students, who shut their hospital to protest its similarly obsolete, understaffed and overcrowded conditions. The orderly Cork strike received quiet encouragement from school authorities, while the Dublin dental hospital experienced a more boisterous student occupation.

In late December 1973 Cork students began circulating petitions calling for the retention of the dental school and the construction of a new hospital. Students collecting signatures in the city's main thoroughfares, with their white clinical coats, becoming a familiar presence throughout January and February. In about ten weeks, students gathered a remarkable thirty-eight thousand signatures – roughly thirty per cent of the city population.

The petition drive underscored perhaps the most convincing argument to retain the school: its importance as a public-health resource for Cork city and the surrounding areas. For decades, the dental hospital had annually treated thousands of patients. For example, the 1968 annual report lists 4,987 first visits; 6,579 general anaesthetics administered; 2,309 X-ray examinations; 66,700 fillings; 121 denture repairs; 897 denture/orthodontic-appliance fittings; 2,868 treatment consultations; and a total of 20,080 attendances. The goodwill built up in the community over the previous sixty years proved decisive to the 'save the school' effort.

In the early months of 1974, the campaign heated up. A media event saw six TDs tour the dental hospital and President McCarthy complain about the minister for education's unwillingness to announce the school's fate. By this time, the 'save the school' campaign had secured the support of the Cork Council of Trade Unions, the Association of Secondary Teachers, Ireland, the Cork branch of the Irish Countrywomen's Association and the Cork Amenity Council. The Southern Health Board proved an influential ally within the public-health sector. The Fianna Fáil Education Committee also endorsed school retention, thus raising it as a national political issue.

The Irish Dental Association endorsed two dental schools for the state, though the stance aroused controversy within the organisation. A vocal Cork proponent was the new IDA president, the charismatic Cork graduate George MacSweeney (BDS 1944). He forcibly promoted the 'two schools' position, arguing for Cork's retention on professional-development and health-care grounds. Beneath a public façade of IDA unity, Cork members believed that Dublin partisans were privately lobbying the government to locate a single dental school in Dublin. It is clear that some IDA members outside of Munster disagreed with the organisation's 'two school' position. The 'one school' idea was not unreasonable, as it would simplify the argument for proper state support of dental education. Indeed, some of these same 'one school' arguments would be made in Cork when the government considered shutting the Dublin dental hospital in the 1980s. However, supporting the closure of one of the two dental schools would be unwise for a national organisation like the IDA, as it would likely produce a damaging internal split between two competing regional interests within the association.

Cork's protests, lobbying and public pressure ultimately beat the government into retreat. In December 1974 Minister for Education Richard Burke announced the state would maintain two dental schools, and would help finance a new Cork dental hospital. The decision featured in Burke's broader plans for higher education, which generated stinging criticism from various institutions and students. Indeed, by this stage the retention of the Cork dental school seems to have become one of the most popular of the minister's besieged higher-education proposals.

BUILDING A HOSPITAL

The new dental-hospital site had been purchased in the 1930s, and designed at the beginning of the 1970s. Construction of what became Cork University Hospital (CUH) began in the summer of 1975. Nationally, the 1973 international oil crisis sent the Irish economy into deep recession, plunging public finances into disarray. Despite the financial fallout, in April 1975 the Department of Education finalised the new dental-hospital design plans. Nervous Cork dental administrators anxiously waited for construction to begin, lest the coffers run dry before ground was broken.

At this critical juncture, in November 1975, a public attack on CUDSH came unexpectedly from the Dublin dental hospital. The staff association of the Dublin dental school issued a scathing report that argued against the state's retention of two dental schools. It criticised the IDA and the Cork dental school for pursuing 'sectional rather than national interests', and denounced 'a misleading comparison of expenditure in the Dublin and Cork

Dental schools'. It further proclaimed that government proposals were 'based on misleading information and not in the best interests of dental education and dentistry'. The staff proposed a single school catering to seventy-five students annually, arguing that keeping two hospitals 'is a serious error that would affect Irish dentistry for a lifetime'. To the Dubliners, the case for selecting the Dublin dental hospital as a single national centre was 'overwhelming'. The report further argued that 'inadequate standards would have been acceptable to UCC' as long as the dental school was retained.

The Dublin dental hospital was in nearly as bad a state as Cork's, but there were no plans to build a new structure in Dublin. Once Cork's new hospital was constructed, the Dublin dental hospital faced possible closure, justified on a rationalisation basis. This drove the Dublin staff to take the extraordinary step of publicly savaging their southern colleagues. Brian Barrett later wrote that 'while one had to sympathise with the frustrating position of the Dublin dental-hospital staff, one would have thought that its staff association would have been using its resources to encourage speedy decisions on the siting and building of the proposed new Dublin dental hospital rather than resurrecting the "one dental school" proposal'. Like a hungry man, the Dublin dental-hospital staff preferred to take the meal of its Cork neighbour rather than demand its own portion.

In the unsettled circumstances, the government became increasingly ambivalent about building the new dental hospital. In April 1976 Minister Burke told the Cork Hospitals Board that owing to precarious public finances, the government could not authorise tender for construction. Within CUDSH, doubts grew about the government's commitment to the institution, raising questions about its long-term viability. The uncertainty made it increasingly difficult to fill staff vacancies, while officials feared a drop in student enrolment.

By now, the dental hospital had entered a terminal stage, with building maintenance downgraded in anticipation of a pending departure for Wilton. The existing building seemed to gradually disintegrate. In the main conservation room, ungainly braces held up the sagging ceiling. When it rained, numerous buckets accommodated steady streams from roof leaks. It was not unknown for loose plaster to drop onto patients and the occasional visiting dignitary. Chairs and equipment were jammed into ungainly spaces, and the basement had become a cave. Brian Barrett described the hospital as 'completely inadequate and grossly over-crowded', and later remarked that it was 'inhuman' to treat patients there. It became increasingly possible that the hospital would be closed for health-and-safety reasons, thus accomplishing what Kaim-Caudle and the HEA could not – shutting the school.

A new round of school lobbying pressured the government to commit to a definite date for hospital construction. The Munster branch of the IDA's Hospital Retention Committee reconvened to coordinate efforts with the dental school. The Southern Health Board lobbied government officials, while students travelled to

Old hospital main conservation room, circa 1980.
<small>Courtesy P.J. Byrne</small>

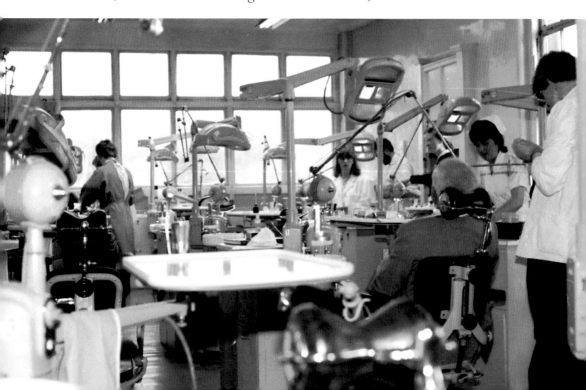

Dublin to picket the Dáil. Gus Healy and Jack Lynch committed Fianna Fáil to building a new hospital, thus placing further pressure on the Fine Gael-led government.

In a case of fortuitous timing, Cork's Peter Barry had succeeded Richard Burke as minister for education. A member of the Cork tea dynasty, Barry recognised the importance of the dental hospital to Cork, but mainly supported the hospital's retention because he 'didn't want to see everything sucked into Dublin'. Within Cabinet he found sympathy for his position among ministers from constituencies outside Dublin. Explaining the Cabinet's deliberations, Barry remarked that when making similar decisions about maintaining existing local institutions or services, some ministers would not be familiar with the intricacies of the debate – instead, they would be inclined to support retention if the decision appeared responsible, did not cost too much, and did not affect their constituency. Retaining the Cork dental hospital ticked all those boxes.

The last key battle was won in early April 1977, when Minister for Education Barry reiterated the government's commitment to a new dental hospital and granted the school permission to negotiate a tender for construction. Contracts were drawn up with John Sisk and Son building contractors, who began the project in November 1977. The following March, 1978, incoming Fianna Fáil minister for labour, Gene Fitzgerald, signed the contracts in front of proud school officials. Like an armistice ceremony, this signalled the final victory in Cork University Dental School and Hospital's nine-year war for survival. Reflecting on the school's roller-coaster ride, Brian Barrett told a reporter: 'We went through a pretty uncertain and unsettling time for a few years.' He did not mention that in the school's darkest days he had begun to quietly circulate his CV, and considered taking up a teaching position in Iran.

Construction took longer than anticipated. Though the new regional-hospital structure opened unofficially in October 1978, the dental hospital would not be ready for another three years.

During that time, students protested against deteriorating hospital conditions at John Redmond Street, this time with less encouragement from school authorities.

Fate gave the school another surprise in the early hours of 14 May 1981. Just as the new hospital prepared to open, fire ravaged the building. A watchman discovered the blaze before it fully gutted the structure, though it still suffered £375,000 in damages. This delayed the hospital's opening for nearly a year.

On 5 March 1982 the chair of the Cork Hospitals Board, Vincent O'Connell, handed over the building keys to the UCC president, Tadhg Ó Ciardha. Dental-school operations shifted over the next months, as the old hospital on John Redmond Street wound down. The official opening took place on 20 June 1983, with Minister of State at the Department of Education Donal Creed cutting the ribbon. Forty-five years after it was first proposed, the Cork university dental school had finally realised its dream of a new hospital.

The Wilton structure was planned to accommodate an annual intake of twenty-five students, up from nineteen. Equipment would meet international standards. To school authorities, the best aspect of the new facility was its co-location with Cork Regional Hospital (now Cork University Hospital), which was attached to the UCC School of Medicine. Connected by a corridor, students could now undertake instruction in pathology and anaesthetics at CUH. The close proximity to the CUH emergency department was greatly appreciated in case of unexpected medical emergency. The access to general anaesthetics expanded oral-surgery options. The hospital library complemented the dental-hospital facility. Lecture theatres, staff canteens and other facilities would be shared. Essentially, the dental hospital was integrated into a modern medical teaching hospital, with all the benefits that implied. Construction cost £3 million, with a third of the total spent on new equipment.

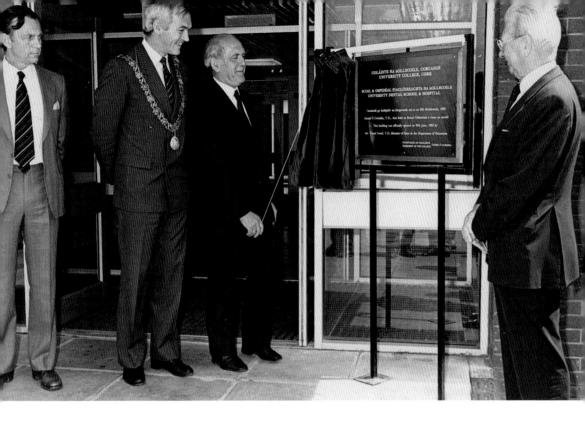

The campaign to save the dental school and build a new hospital depended on support received at an institutional, local and national level. School staff members Louis Buckley, Finbarr Corkery, Finbarr O'Sullivan and many others lobbied consistently on behalf of CUDSH. Within the school administration, the key figure was Brian Barrett, who successfully built a broad and effective alliance of advocates. Tim Riordan's Munster IDA committee likewise merited significant credit, as did two local TDs, Gus Healy and Peter Barry. The people of Cork proved the most powerful constituency in favour of retaining the dental school, and their voice was ultimately heard by the government. All deserved recognition for their tremendous service to CUDSH during its darkest hour. Perhaps the most unique contribution came from the students themselves, who sacrificed their time over a number of years.

The student effort can be attributed to a strong student society, good peer leadership (offered by such members as Tom Boland,

Opening of the new Cork University Dental School and Hospital, 1983: (left to right) B. Barrett, Lord Mayor H. Coveney, Minister of State D. Creed, UCC President T. O'Ciardha.
Courtesy Brian Barrett

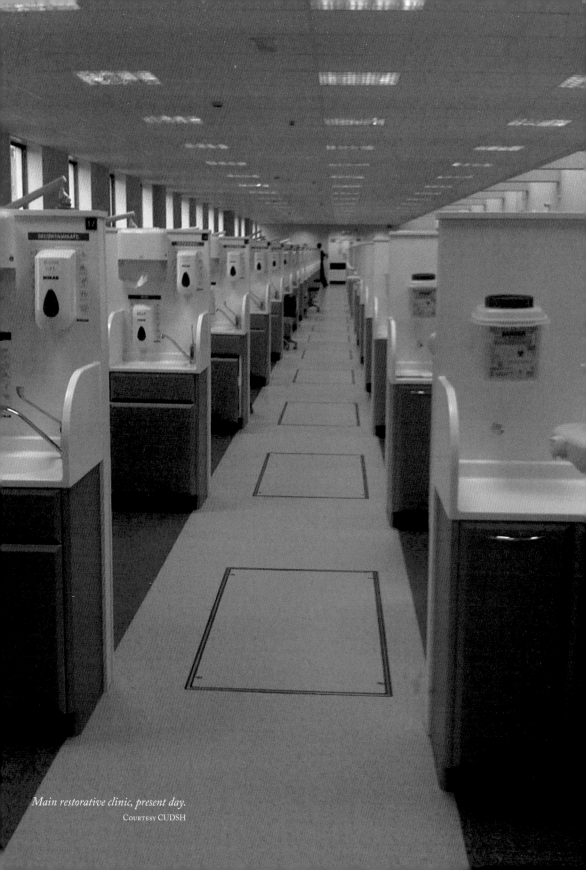

Main restorative clinic, present day.
COURTESY CUDSH

Seán Russell, Noel Walsh, Dan Finn and others) and a dedicated student body. In this period of Irish history, such grass-roots organisation was not uncommon; indeed, many citizens considered participation in protests and strikes a social responsibility rather than a burden. Ultimately, the school owes a debt of gratitude to those students who laboured long hours in the cold and rain, or travelled to Dublin to ensure the institution survived for those following behind them. Their achievement was substantial. With the construction of a new hospital, the Cork university dental school entered a new era as a modern centre of training, scholarship and research.

5

THE NEW DENTAL SCHOOL & HOSPITAL, 1983 TO PRESENT

----

*T*HE opening of the new dental hospital ushered in a new era in the Cork University Dental School and Hospital. Individual degree programmes and teaching departments, often lingering in the embryonic stage, received enough resources to flourish. Scholarship improved, clinical services expanded, and the student-body composition altered. Changes became so significant and widespread that they should be considered individually rather than chronologically.

GOVERNANCE

Cork University Dental School and Hospital.
COURTESY CUDSH

UCC formally took over management of the Cork dental hospital from the North Infirmary governing body in 1968. CUDSH later became one of the six schools comprising UCC's College of Medicine and Health. The dental hospital is essentially self-governed by the CUDSH faculty, answering to University College Cork. This rare management arrangement worked well while the

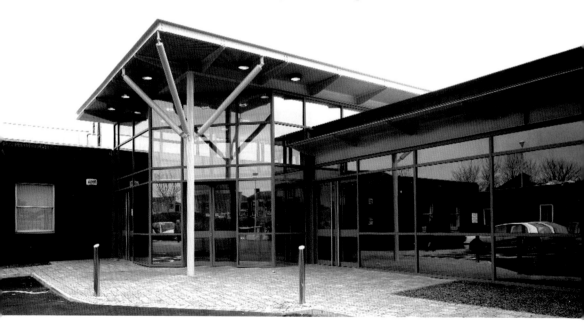

school remained relatively small, but the growth of the past two decades has made it more cumbersome.

The head of CUDSH has never been an easy role. The Cork Dental School and Hospital's tripartite mission of teaching, service and research usually makes it impossible to fully satisfy the various constituencies inside and outside CUDSH. As such, the head of school must possess professional proficiency and personal tact, along with strong reserves of inner strength. Fortunately, CUDSH has been blessed with sound leadership throughout the modern era.

Professor Brian Barrett assumed the title of director of dental studies when he was appointed to the school in 1963, essentially renaming the position of school dean. Professor Barrett remained head of the school for the next twenty years during a very successful tenure that included the 'save the school' campaign. He was replaced in 1991 by Professor Louis Buckley (BDS 1957), a popular figure among the dental-nursing and clinical-teaching staff. Beyond his term as head of school, Louis should be remembered for establishing Cork's dental-nursing and dental-hygienists training programmes. Louis was followed by Professor Denis O'Mullane (BDS 1958), an international authority on water fluoridation, an author of more than 150 peer-reviewed articles, and one of Ireland's most accomplished dental scholars. Among his many contributions to the school was establishing the Oral Health Services Research Centre and mentoring a generation of dental academics. Professor Robbie McConnell, chair of Restorative Dentistry, succeeded Professor O'Mullane in 1998, and served until 2006. While head of school, he refurbished the hospital and recruited specialist staff, who in turn provided greater community-health services. A well-liked teacher and skilled administrator, he oversaw the vertical integration of the school curriculum and the school's ascension into UCC's newly established College of Medicine and Health. Professor Finbarr Allen (BDS 1988) followed Professor McConnell, and greatly expanded research

GEORGE MacSWEENEY: 'IT'S ALL IN THE HANDS, YOU KNOW'

One of the Cork dental school's most colourful graduates was George MacSweeney. Born in 1917 to a chemist who operated a shop on Patrick Street, MacSweeney attended Christian Brothers College. At an early age he developed a love of music, and learned piano at the Cork School of Music. Thereafter he devoted himself to two passions: dentistry and music.

After qualifying from the Cork dental school in 1944, MacSweeney went into private practice in Macroom, County Cork. He later joined the public dental service on the Isle of Man, which led to his appointment as chief dental surgeon with the Cork Health Authority. In that role he expanded rural dental services, reaching many members of the public for the first time. He became a vocal advocate of oral-disease prevention, and supported water-fluoridation initiatives undertaken in County Cork. In 1965 George received a public-health diploma from Boston University, and was awarded a foundation fellowship by the dentistry faculty of the RCSI. Now chief dental officer for the city and county of Cork, his department purchased and equipped a mobile home to bring dental clinics to remote parts of the county. By the end of the decade, George was managing public dental-health services in counties Cork and Kerry. In 1973 he was elected president of the Irish Dental Association, its first president selected from the public service. His tenure coincided with Cork's 'save the school' campaign. George acted as an important advocate for CUDSH, mobilising IDA members in the school's defence and using his position to argue for retention of two dental schools on health-care and professional grounds.

Beyond dentistry, George MacSweeney was a noted musical entertainer locally and nationally. While studying at CUDSH by day, George played gigs at night. An accomplished keyboard player, he was well known for his skill with the piano accordion. He and his accordion became regulars at the Sunday-night variety shows held in Cork Opera House, and he was often sent onstage to restore order in between acts when crowds grew too boisterous (they occasionally disrupted indulgent opera singers with whistling or by rolling beer bottles down the aisles). He subsequently starred in his own weekly radio programme, *At Home with George MacSweeney*, initially broadcast from the old Cork women's gaol. The musical-variety show remained a popular fixture on RTÉ throughout the 1940s and early 1950s.

George MacSweeney.
COURTESY
GEORGE MACSWEENEY JNR.

MacSweeney retained a special affection for the cinema organ. He frequently practised on the Savoy Cinema organ, which he played every year for the duration of the Cork Film Festival. This service gave rise to one of his favourite stories. During a film-festival appearance by the British actor Peter Cushing (of Dracula and Sherlock Holmes fame), organisers sent word to MacSweeney that Mr Cushing needed assistance with a dislodged bridge. When MacSweeney promptly fixed the problem, the actor expressed amazement that an organist could possess such dental dexterity. It's all in the hands, you know', George supposedly replied. He remained a devoted member of the Cinema Organ Society, and still travelled to their gatherings in Britain after his retirement from the public-health service in 1982.

George MacSweeney died in 2005. He was a loyal friend of the Cork dental school, and one of its effervescent personalities

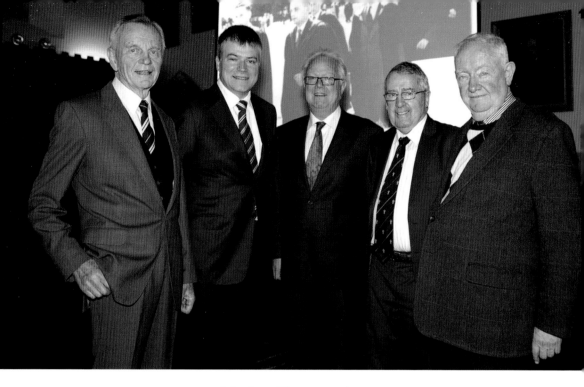

Former school deans at CUDSH centenary celebration, March 2013: (left to right) professors Brian Barrett, Finbarr Allen, Robbie McConnell, Denis O'Mullane, Louis Buckley.

Courtesy Tomás Tyner, UCC

outputs and funding. This was in keeping with his record as one of Ireland's top dental researchers, having authored three monographs and numerous articles. He enjoys close personal connections with CUDSH through his father Vincent Allen (BDS 1959), and wife and classmate Dr Edith Allen (née Finn), currently the school's third-year coordinator. Professor Allen's tenure concluded during the school's 2013 centenary, an anniversary he embraced and which resulted in this book. His successor, Professor Martin Kinirons (BDS 1976), boasts an equally strong record of scholarship, having published over 120 peer-reviewed articles. Like his predecessors, Professors Allen, McConnell, O'Mullane and Buckley, Dr Kinirons obtained a Ph.D. and built an impressive research portfolio.

INTERNATIONAL STUDENTS

Up until 1980, the Cork student body was almost exclusively native-born Irish. That began to change later in the decade, and especially in the 1990s. International students came primarily from developing countries in Africa and the Middle East. They introduced racial and cultural diversity to the school and hospital at a time when multiculturalism was still largely unknown in Ireland. Visiting students also had to navigate the cultural complexities of treating patients who behaved differently than those in their native country, as well as learning to decipher the Cork accent. Staff found the international students to be of a generally high standard and it was noted that they took their studies seriously. An international officer was appointed – Mary Hall (married to Professor John Hall of the Department of Physiology) – as a point of contact for these students, and to act as a cultural and educational liaison.

The first wave of international students was dominated by those coming from the Middle East, especially Kuwait, Oman and the United Arab Emirates. Students from Malaysia subsequently began to register at CUDSH, along with many from Botswana. This traffic has not been one-way, as a number of Cork faculty members have travelled to the Middle East to serve as consultants and externs for the emerging dental-education system there. Cork graduate Professor Robin O'Sullivan has become a major figure in dental medical education, first in Kuwait and currently in Bahrain.

International students pay full fees at the Cork dental school. Their numbers have risen steadily in recent years, following broader Irish university trends, especially within the medical faculties. Recently, students from Canada and the United States have been drawn to Cork. The exchange with Canada was bolstered in 2012 by the former head of school, Professor Robbie McConnell, acting on behalf of the Dental Council of Ireland. He successfully negotiated with the Commission of Dental Accreditation of Canada to recognise the Irish dental qualification there. Canadian and Irish students can now practise in Canada after receiving a BDS from CUDSH, strengthening this transatlantic link. Overall, international students today comprise nearly a third of BDS graduates, stretching the Cork dental-school community far beyond the shores of Ireland.

PART-TIME STAFF

Since the school's foundation, the pay and status of the part-time teaching staff has been an ongoing concern, resulting twice in the withdrawal of their labour. These appear to have been the only such strikes by academic staff in UCC history. While the first stoppage in 1926 lasted only a few days, the second in 1998 carried on for most of a year.

CUDSH has always relied on part-time instructors to undertake chair and floor teaching duties. However, historically these staff members were not recognised as university employees. Most did not teach for financial reasons, as they gave up lucrative time from their practice to be paid very low rates for three-hour sessions at the dental hospital. Teachers usually made the sacrifice in order to continue their education, to give something back to the discipline, to maintain their skills, for the joy of teaching, and for the collegiality of the school. Yet the lack of university recognition of their service grated on staff members. Their hourly pay rate was low by anyone's standards, and they also failed to receive pension contributions, holiday pay, sick pay, maternity leave or special payment for teaching courses.

These benefits fell within the remit of the UCC personnel department, beyond the control of CUDSH. Approaches to the university were repeatedly rebuffed, and frustration built up over a number of years. According to strike leader Noel Walsh, 'our goodwill was stretched beyond endurance' as the university displayed 'utter, utter disregard for what we were doing' as teachers. The newly appointed school dean, Denis O'Mullane, agreed with the part-time-staff grievances but had little power to resolve the dispute. Ultimately, the staff withdrew their services from the hospital. (They did not picket the location as they did not have official union representation.) The dispute dragged on for months, and the maintenance of teaching rotas challenged CUDSH authorities. Only when the hospital faced possible closure was a settlement reached. Essentially, UCC agreed to all the staff demands, which university administrators retrospectively regarded as entirely reasonable. At long last, the part-time teaching staff, who had been the bedrock of CUDSH since its foundation, received some of the recognition they richly deserved. It was unfortunate that it only came about as a result of a bitter strike that left bad blood within the school for some years afterwards.

RESTORATIVE DENTISTRY & GERODONTOLOGY

During the last quarter-century, Irish oral health has steadily improved. Dramatic declines in adult tooth loss have transformed dental education and dental treatment at CUDSH. Until the 1990s, older adult dental treatment focused on extractions and dentures. This emphasis carried over into student instruction, with students spending a full year learning to fabricate dentures (working alongside trainee dental technicians from 1983 to 1990) and attending a final-year session in prosthetic dentistry. Gradually, dentistry shifted away from extraction and towards preservation of natural teeth. Improved materials for dental bonding (to teeth) have further expanded treatment options. This research area has been strong in Cork since Bill McCullough's appointment to the school's chair in prosthetic dentistry in 1969. His work on castable glass ceramics is still regarded as seminal in the field of ceramic restoration. Dr Noel Ray, lecturer in dental materials, further contributed to bonding research, as has Professor Robbie McConnell (head of the Department of Restorative Dentistry from 1995 to 2000, and head of school from 2000 to 2006). CUDSH students now learn minimally invasive dentistry and the use of adhesive techniques for cavity restoration, replacing amalgam as a restorative material.

CUDSH was an early advocate of the use of dental implants. In the early 1980s, researchers coined the term 'osseointegration' to

NOEL WALSH:
TEACHER & ACTIVIST

James Noel Walsh was born in Ballintemple, Cork, in 1942, and educated at Presentation Brothers College. After his Leaving Cert, he spent five years working in the insurance business with Norwich Union. He surprised his employers by resigning to study dentistry at UCC as a mature student. It was a decision he never regretted.

At UCC, Noel took an active role in student politics, serving on the Comhairle Teacthi Na Mac Léinn, the forerunner of the Student Union. He played a pivotal role as auditor of the Cork Dental Student Society during the early stages of the battle to save the school. One of his coups was convincing Taoiseach Jack Lynch to accept a dinner invitation from the Student Society, in order to put before him the case for retaining dentistry. Noel also helped establish the Irish Dental Students' Association, becoming its first president. Along the way, he married his classmate Philomena Floyd (BDS 1972), and the two set up practice, first in Britain and then in Wexford, before returning to Blackrock, Cork.

A natural leader, Noel became active in the Irish Dental Association. His positions with the IDA's Munster branch eventually led to his election as IDA president in 1991. During his term, he came under fire from Dublin dental-school advocates, who accused him of undermining their efforts to secure a new school and hospital. This was a misperception based primarily on his Cork pedigree. In fact, Noel always supported the IDA's 'two school policy', believing competition was healthy for Irish dentistry, as it allowed different ideas and practices to develop within the two schools.

In 1978 he joined the part-time clinical-teaching staff at CUDSH, initially commuting once a week from Wexford, before settling again in Cork. Within school history, Noel should be credited with a long but successful campaign to secure full benefits for the part-time teaching staff, including holiday and sick pay,

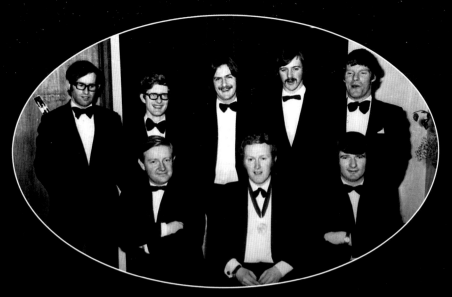

Cork dental students committee Dental Ball, Imperial Hotel, Cork, 1972:
(back, left to right) C. O'Loughlin, N. O'Neill, D. Murray, M. Quinlivan, R. O'Neill;
(front, left to right) L. Buckley, Noel Walsh, J. Collins.

maternity leave and access to the pension scheme. Essentially, he helped
fundamentally alter the school's approach to its part-time clinical staff, which
previously had frequently been perceived as filling hours while they built
up their personal practice. Instead, Noel envisioned the position as offering
another career pathway into dental education.

Noel eventually led his part-time colleagues out on strike, which proved
trying to both sides. Though the struggle lasted longer than anticipated,
it ended with a full victory for the staff. The strike divided part-time and
tenured staff, but even Noel's opponents recognised his fundamental honesty
and integrity, which helped reduce bad feelings.

Ultimately, Noel spent thirty years on CUDSH's clinical-teaching staff.
He remained popular among students, who appreciated his patience and
willingness to speak up for anyone he felt was being treated unfairly. That
kind of courage is a rare and valued commodity in any institution.

For his part, Noel reflected that his tenure at CUDSH had its ups and
downs. He always appreciated his first mentor, Professor Louis Buckley,
who became his lifelong friend. After retiring from the school in 2008, Noel
continued in his Blackrock practice. Today, much of his time is spent with
his beloved Cork Constitution Rugby Club, which he served as president in
2002–03. It would appear that his leadership was recognised by more than
one storied institution.

describe a new phenomenon whereby allogenic materials (which integrate with living tissue) could be grafted to replace missing teeth. Dr Gerry Buckley and Dr Tony Aherne studied this breakthrough technique in Sweden during the mid-1980s, and brought it to Cork. Within a few years, Dr Buckley and his colleague Professor Duncan Sleeman were offering complex dental-implant treatments to patients. This led to the establishment of a dedicated dental-implant assessment clinic, currently headed by Professor Duncan Sleeman and Professor Finbarr Allen. The internationally renowned Straumann and Nobel Biocare dental-implant companies recognise CUDSH as an implantology training centre, and both companies have supported training for selected Cork staff and students.

The ageing phenomenon (people living longer) coupled with greater tooth retention has led to the emergence of the new discipline of gerodontology, which responds to clinical issues among elderly patients. Following the appointment of Dr Frank Burke in 1998, the dental-school teaching programme addressed cross-disciplinary management of older patients. Students received dedicated teaching in such areas as tooth-wear management, endodontics for the elderly, and treatment of the medically compromised patient. Oral care of the elderly has become a major research area within CUDSH, which is now recognised internationally in the field. For over a decade, Cork researchers have conducted clinical trials of preventive and treatment strategies for the elderly, and evaluated minimally invasive dentistry in terms of quality-of-life impact, cost and clinical effectiveness. Dr Gerry McKenna (lecturer in prosthodontics and oral rehabilitation, and coordinator of the fourth-year BDS programme) won the Hatton Senior Clinical Award at the International Association for Dental Research meeting in 2012, the first Irish winner of this prestigious international competition. Awarded a doctorate by UCC in 2012, Dr McKenna has shown that restoration of shortened dental arches with adhesive-fixed bridgework is more cost-effective than the provision of removable partial dentures in elderly patients. His colleague, Professor Finbarr Allen, received the Distinguished Scientist Award from the International Association for Dental Research (IADR) in 2011 in recognition of his research career in geriatric oral health, which includes one hundred peer-reviewed articles. In 2012 Professor Allen gave the keynote address at the IADR annual meeting in Brazil.

Together, the aforementioned have an enviable record that has carried on from the early work of Bill McCullough.

DENTAL SURGERY

Following the appointment of Professor Gordon Russell in 1963, the dental-surgery academic undergraduate programme expanded to include teaching in oral medicine. Clinical treatment occurred within the dental hospital, while out-of-hours emergencies were treated in the North Infirmary. The teaching of minor oral surgery grew substantially in the 1970s after the arrival of Dr Finbarr Corkery.

In the 1990s students received instruction in facial-trauma surgery, which was a speciality of the newly appointed Dr Conor O'Brien. Under the auspices of the Mid-Western Health Board, Dr O'Brien also conducted monthly minor-oral-surgery clinics outside Cork – in Limerick and Clonmel – assisted by dental nurse Mary McCarthy (who married Barry Johnson). These clinics undertook oral-surgical procedures and followed up on trauma cases previously treated in the CUDSH Oral Surgery Department.

The new dental hospital offered far superior facilities for surgical treatment, which resulted in a rapid growth of in-patient orthognathic (jaw surgery) cases. The addition of Professor Duncan Sleeman to the school led to the development of oral and maxillofacial surgical services during the 1990s. This multifaceted oral-surgery programme now includes postgraduate training programmes. By the early 2000s, a new generation of students enjoyed expanded teaching and clinical services in oral medicine under Dr Christine McCreery, and in dental radiology under Dr Donal McDonnell. The recent establishment of the postgraduate D.Clin.Dent. (Oral Surgery) diploma replicates similar trends in other departments. Two such graduates were conferred in 2013: Dr Emma Warren and Dr Michael McAuliffe. The multitude of surgery options at CUDSH would have been inconceivable just a few decades before.

ORAL RADIOLOGY

Radiology has progressed considerably since Israel Scher brought the first X-ray machine to Cork in 1923. Developments in film type, holding devices and machine speed have reduced radiation exposure. Digital-imaging systems introduced in the 1980s improved sensor size, generated finer image quality, and reduced costs of imaging. At the same time, new European Economic Community (now European Union) health-care directives required the licensing and testing of radiology equipment, the retention and auditing of records, and investigations of radiographic incidents. These changes necessitated sophisticated training of operators and support staff, whose ranks included qualified dental nurses and hygienists.

The dental schools in Dublin and Cork have combined forces under the National Dental Nurse Training Programme of Ireland. Dental nurses and hygienists receive instruction in all aspects of intraoral and panoramic radiology, with the didactic component provided in the School of Medicine and Medical Science, University College Dublin, in collaboration with the state's two dental schools.

Oral radiology (or oral and maxillofacial radiology) is a recognised speciality in many countries, and was conducted in Cork by

Dr Donal McDonnell until his retirement in 2011. The majority of dental images are still bitewings, periapicals and panoramics, reflecting the common dental conditions of caries, periodontal disease, unerupted teeth and dental anomalies. State-of-the-art imaging can be achieved through such techniques as cone beam computerised tomography (CBCT), ultrasound (US) and magnetic resonance imaging (MRI). These help maxillofacial surgeons and implantologists manage trauma, tumours and complicated implant cases. Orthodontists and surgeons can better plan orthognathic cases via three-dimensional imaging. There is an increasing use of CBCT (for example, in endodontics) for conditions affecting the dentition. Such facilities are available in Cork University Hospital, with CUDSH's clinical-graduate programme enjoying access to each technique.

ORAL MEDICINE

Oral medicine is a dental speciality located at the interface between dentistry and medicine, treating conditions primarily without surgery. Many oral-medicine specialists have dental and medical qualifications, although specialist training no longer requires a medical degree. Oral medicine arrived as a full-time speciality in Cork with the appointment of Dr Christine McCreery in 2002 (it had previously been taught as a subject by Gordon Russell, in addition to his other duties). She remains one of the state's three oral-medicine consultants.

Dr McCreery's department operates with a dedicated nurse and rotating junior staff in training positions. In recent years, four to five clinics have been held weekly, with patient referrals stretching from Galway to Wexford. Undergraduate students rotate through all of the oral-medicine clinics, taking patient histories and observing some oral-mucosal and other related conditions, such as xerostomia. Treatment requires regular liaisons with specialists in such fields as dermatology, gastroenterology, immunology and oncology. The department's research profile has expanded in recent years through the addition of clinical research-fellow posts. Dr Richeal Ní Ríordáin (BDS 2002, Ph.D. 2011) was the department's first clinical fellow (a talented violinist, she also formerly led the violin section of the Cork Symphony Orchestra, and is currently studying medicine in London). Oral medicine has made significant strides in the decades since its establishment, and is now recognised as a potential growth field within CUDSH.

PREVENTIVE & PAEDIATRIC DENTISTRY

The teaching of preventive and paediatric dentistry began as a separate subject in 1966. The corresponding department enjoyed strong leadership from its founder Chris Collins (1966–76), which was continued by his successors, Dr Jim Mageean (1976–78), Dr Tim Holland (1978–82), Professor Denis O'Mullane (1982–2003) and Professor Martin Kinirons (2004 to present). During that time, the department has undertaken several innovative initiatives that have delivered critical public-health services directly to the public.

Perhaps the department's most interesting project was the Specialist Unit for Treatment of People with Severe Disabilities. A 1978 Department of Health report called for the establishment of special dental units to treat people with mental and physical disabilities, whose needs had been previously neglected. At CUDSH, this service was established by Dr Tim Holland through the Department of Preventive and Paediatric Dentistry, collaborating with the Southern Health Board to provide both primary and secondary care to these patients.

The Specialist Unit under Dr Holland operated in the new Cork University Hospital (CUH), with its facilities consisting of an operating theatre, an immediate recovery area and a day-stay ward.

An anaesthetist, a dentist, a dental-surgery assistant and three staff nurses comprised the core staff. When it opened in 1984, the unit staff members were Dr Tim Holland (dental consultant), Dr Peter Kennefick (consulting anaesthetist), Kathryn Neville (dental nurse), and Irene O'Mahony, Karen Kelleher and Bernie Spain (staff nurses). Patient referrals came via institutions for whom the department had assumed responsibility, as well as from Health Board staff and general practitioners throughout the Southern, South-Eastern, and Mid-Western regions. The unit opened in early 1984, treating two patients with severe disabilities per week. Dental students regularly observed the proceedings, offering the undergraduates a valuable learning experience. From 1997 to 2007, the Specialist Unit completed seven hundred courses of treatment for patients across multiple age ranges. The Specialist Unit's success in this period underlines the state's growing awareness of its institutional population, as well as CUDSH's ongoing commitment to public health. Following a 2007 service agreement between the Health Service Executive (HSE) and CUDSH, treatment in the Specialist Unit for patients up to the age of sixteen years has been carried out through the Department of Preventive and Paediatric Dentistry. The current consultant in charge is Professor Martin Kinirons, and the HSE dental surgeons operating the unit are Dr Fiona Graham and Dr Caroline Hartnett. Patients over the age of sixteen are treated in the same unit during a separate anaesthetic session by Dr Patrick Quinn, senior clinical dental surgeon HSE, under the direction of Dr Chris Cotter, HSE consultant in oral and maxillofacial surgery.

During the early 1980s, the department sought to expose students to working conditions beyond the dental hospital. Professor Denis O'Mullane and Dr Tim Holland secured agreement from the Southern Health Board to allow students to complete some of their clinical training at Health Board dental clinics in Cork city. Final-year students spent one three-hour session per month treating patients at the inner-city Health Board dental clinics at St Finbarr's Hospital and at Grattan Street. Supervision of training in these clinics was provided by Health Board dental staff, primarily Dr Kevin Quinlan at St Finbarr's and Dr Colm Bell at Grattan Street. Prior to starting the programme, Dr Quinlan and Dr Bell obtained a year of teaching experience in the department's teaching clinics.

A programme to provide dental care for Cork schoolchildren at the old dental hospital commenced in 1923 and ended in 1938, following the establishment of a dental clinic at Cork City Hall. Subsequently, children attended the dental hospital on a demand-only basis. In 1991, however, following discussions with the Southern Health Board, the Department of Preventive and Paediatric Dentistry began treating Cork schoolchildren. The department provided comprehensive dental care to children attending ten schools (Gaelscoil Uí Riada, Scoil Therese, Scoil an Spioraid Naoimh (boys and girls), St Catherine's, Canovee, Cloghroe, Coachford, Dripsey and Kilmurray). Dental care was carried out by third-year and final-year clinical students under supervision, with more-complex treatments undertaken by junior and consultant staff. This initiative gave students a wide experience caring for diverse paediatric patients.

At this same time, the department undertook primary and secondary care for three institutions catering for people with mental and physical disabilities: at St Patrick's (Upton, County Cork), St Mary's (Rochestown, County Cork) and the Children's Assessment and Treatment Centre (Cork city). The department also treated special-needs students at the School of the Divine Child (Lavanagh Centre, Cork). The initiative added an important dimension to undergraduate dental training while also providing a critical service to a historically marginalised segment of Irish society.

ORTHODONTICS

In 1916 the first question on orthodontics appeared in a Cork BDS exam paper. Orthodontic questions regularly showed up on dental-surgery and/or mechanical-dentistry BDS exam papers in ensuing years, but there was no separate paper on orthodontics. The dedicated teaching of orthodontics appears to have started in 1938, when the school appointed E. Sheldon Friel as a part-time lecturer in orthodontics. At that time, Friel taught at TCD, and commuted to Cork for his lectures. He was subsequently appointed professor of orthodontics at TCD in 1941, the first such position in Europe (for a number of years, Friel remained the only orthodontics professor in Britain or Ireland). In 1950 Dr Rodney Dockrell succeeded Friel as visiting lecturer in orthodontics at Cork, which led to the appearance of the first BDS paper devoted to orthodontics. Dockrell subsequently became professor of orthodontics and school dean at TCD, but he continued to teach and examine at Cork until the appointment of Professor Mary Hegarty in 1964.

Beyond Professor Hegarty's status as the first female chair in the school, she was one of the longest-serving faculty members. Two of Professor Hegarty's children later joined the dental profession: Anne Hegarty (BDS 1987), a specialist in restorative dentistry, and David Hegarty (BDS 1990), a consultant orthodontist. The department's clinical-teaching staff members were all part-time: Dr Claire Barry, Dr Bridget Dineen, Dr Owen Crotty, Dr John Buckley and Dr Donal Cahill. Its visiting consultants were Dr Dan Counihan, Dr William Murphy and Dr Seamus Keating.

Patient referrals for opinion and treatment came from general dental practitioners, community dental surgeons, medical consultants and from within the dental hospital. For many years, the Dental Hospital Orthodontic Department provided the principal orthodontic service to children and adults in the Munster region. The scheme was closely linked to clinical-teaching programmes, and provided material for both clinical teaching and research.

Postgraduate orthodontic-training programmes were also initiated. Successive junior hospital staff and dental surgeons from the Health Boards and general practice received academic and clinical training in preparation for the professional postgraduate examinations of the Royal Colleges of Surgeons. Among them were Dr Bridget Dineen, Dr Noel Power and Dr Claire Barry, each of whom attained the Dip. Orth. RCS (Eng.). Dr Dan Counihan also went on to complete a higher-training programme to consultant level in the UK. In technical training, instructor Charles Foley received a distinction in the Advanced Certificate in Orthodontics, London City and Guilds for dental craftsmen. His son John (BDS 1983) is currently a member of the part-time teaching staff.

Professor Declan Millett succeeded Professor Hegarty as professor of orthodontics in 2003. By that time, orthodontics had become a national political issue, which resulted in an initiative to train specialist orthodontists in Cork. Under Professor Millett, the department received substantial financial assistance from the HSE (which continues today), and built a new clinical facility to deliver a postgraduate programme in orthodontics (D.Clin.Dent.). Additional laboratory and teaching areas were also created.

The first intake of four students commenced in October 2006. The programme is Ireland's first taught doctorate programme in orthodontics, and is approved by the Irish Committee for Specialist Training in Dentistry of the Royal College of Surgeons. Graduates are eligible for inclusion on the Specialist List in Orthodontics held by the Dental Council, and the programme also meets the educational requirements for membership examinations of the Royal Colleges of Surgeons.

The new Orthodontic Unit treats patients from the north Cork area of the HSE (South). Referred patients are assessed with the Index of Orthodontic Treatment Need (IOTN), with only those meeting HSE eligibility criteria receiving treatment. Orthodontic assessments are undertaken mainly by undergraduate

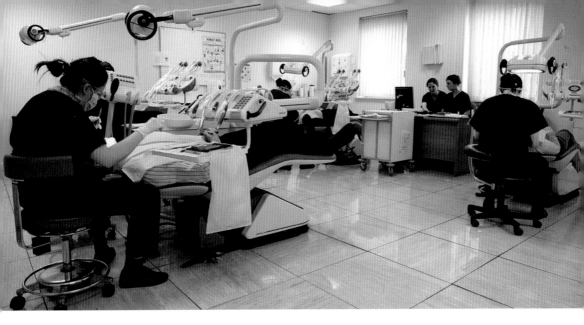

Main clinic,
School of Dental Hygiene.
COURTESY CUDSH

or postgraduate dental students acting under the supervision of a consultant/specialist calibrated in IOTN. Postgraduate orthodontic-programme students treat these patients, thus directly linking HSE clinical care with student training. The D.Clin.Dent. degree also entails a research component, which has produced some fascinating projects.

The current members of staff in the Orthodontic Unit consist of Professor Declan Millett, Dr Denis Field (lecturer/consultant), Dr Patricia McDermott (lecturer/specialist) and Mr John Brown (lecturer in dental technology, orthodontics).

DENTAL NURSING & DENTAL HYGIENE

Dentists in the early twentieth century employed assistants to help treat patients. The first formal staff-training programmes commenced in Britain during the 1930s, and the British Dental Nurses and Assistants Examining Board was founded in 1943. Recognising Ireland's deficiency in this regard, Professor Louis Buckley launched a dental-nurse training programme at CUDSH nearly thirty years later, the first in Ireland.

Initial dental-nurse training was conducted in the old dental hospital, with the first class in 1971 comprised of part-time

KATHRYN NEVILLE: DENTAL NURSE, MANAGER & HOSPITAL ADMINISTRATOR

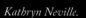

Kathryn Neville.

During Kathryn Neville's twenty-five-year service in the CUDSH, she developed strong management and people skills, which have helped her find additional career success in university administration.

Kathryn joined the CUDSH as a trainee dental nurse in 1979, one of the last groups of students to cycle through the old hospital on John Redmond Street. Following her two-year training programme, she worked mainly in the children's department. After the move to the new hospital at Wilton, Kathryn was instrumental in helping Dr Tim Holland establish his specialist unit to provide care for adults and children with special needs in the Munster area. Bright, energetic and highly efficient, she became an invaluable member of the team.

Continuing her education, Kathryn obtained a BA in English and a postgraduate diploma in computer science. She then joined the Oral Health Services Research Centre as a project manager. In this period, she worked on a number of EU-funded research projects requiring close collaboration with European universities. Many of the world's leading health-care companies participated in industry-funded projects, which often utilised a different skill set. The establishment of, and adherence to, protocols, standards, best practices and milestones brought a healthy scrutiny and robustness to her work. Now possessing diverse professional experience, Kathryn completed a Master in Business Administration (MBA). She subsequently became the manager of the Oral Health Services Research Centre, overseeing its growth from a single office to the established, internationally recognised enterprise it is today.

In 1998 Kathryn was promoted to manager of Cork University

Dental School and Hospital. Working initially with Professor Denis O'Mullane and, later, with Professor Robert McConnell, she helped secure funding for a refurbishment of the hospital interior, and oversaw the installation of new dental chairs, sterilisers, simulation units and a new orthodontic extension. During her tenure, she emphasised the school's spirit of service to patients and students, setting and achieving a high standard in the process. One of her initiatives was the installation of a simple patient-feedback system. She took pride in the fact that positive comments overwhelmingly outnumbered the negative.

In 2007 Kathryn left the familiar confines of CUDSH for the new Cork University Maternity Hospital, where she managed the Department of Obstetrics and Gynaecology. While there, the hospital opened Ireland's first purpose-built, integrated research-and-clinical centre devoted to women's health and reproduction. Kathryn worked to combine clinical care with research and teaching, working closely with Professor John Higgins in the process. This led to her joining the minister for health's project team that established hospital groups in Ireland, one of the most influential health-care initiatives undertaken in recent years. In 2009 Kathryn became manager of the College of Medicine and Health at UCC. Currently, she retains overall responsibility for the delivery of administrative support services within the college. She oversees the formulation and implementation of its strategic plan, directs resource planning, works with the university's Human Resource and Finance departments, and ensures efficient and effective administration within the college.

Throughout her career, Kathryn Neville has proved herself a master of detail, while demonstrating an institutional loyalty that inspires those around her. Those who recall her early years in the dental hospital have observed with satisfaction her many successes since leaving the dental school. Dentistry's loss has been the wider university's gain.

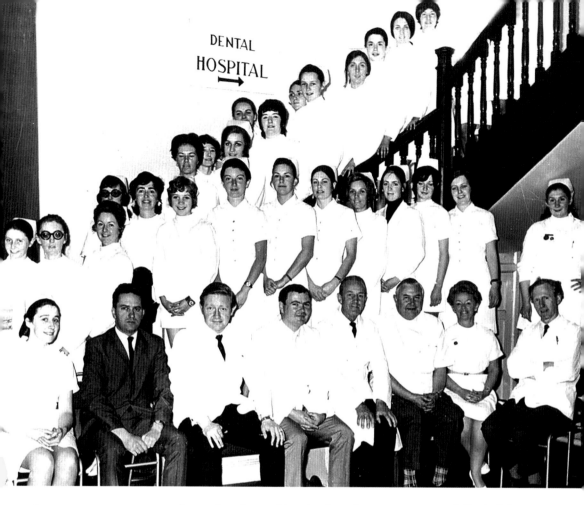

DENTAL HOSPITAL →

Graduation of first dental nursing class, 1971, entrance to old dental hospital, John Redmond Street.

COURTESY CUDSH

students already working in dental practices around Cork. Mary Coughlan filled the role of tutor, until she was succeeded by Eilish O'Mahony. A dedicated and inspired leader, Ms O'Mahony developed the course over the next twenty years. In recognition of her important contributions to CUDSH, the Eilish O'Mahony Award is now given to the top dental-nursing student. The dental-nursing qualification requires eighteen months of study, and usually graduates thirty-five to forty nurses.

In 2004 the National Dental Nurse Training Programme of Ireland, jointly operated by the Cork and Dublin dental schools, began offering remote dental-nursing education. Students outside Cork and Dublin receive lectures and tutorials delivered by a combination of teaching methodologies, including video conferencing. Since 2009 CUDSH has given student nurses the option of gaining their clinical experience within the Cork dental hospital rather than as trainee nurses in private practices. They attend each clinic for a number of weeks on a rotational basis, becoming familiar with all aspects of clinical dentistry. Currently, CUDSH has thirty-two dental-nursing students undertaking a diploma on-site, and an additional ten at Waterford Institute of Technology outreach centre.

Like dental nursing, the training of dental hygienists began in Ireland decades after it had become an international norm. The role calls for a clinical professional to educate patients in oral health, working in collaboration with a dental team directed by the dentist. CUDSH opened the purpose-built School of Dental Hygiene in 1993, with Professor Buckley acting as its first director and Anne O'Keeffe as tutor. The initial graduates were Anne Holohan, Karen Lehane, Susan O'Mahony and Zita White. Anne Holohan now serves on the school's teaching staff (her husband Martin has been

Dental nurse graduation, 1998: (left to right) G. Crowley, L. Martin, H. McAuliffe, S. Fennell, E. Carroll, S. Cronin.
Courtesy CUDSH

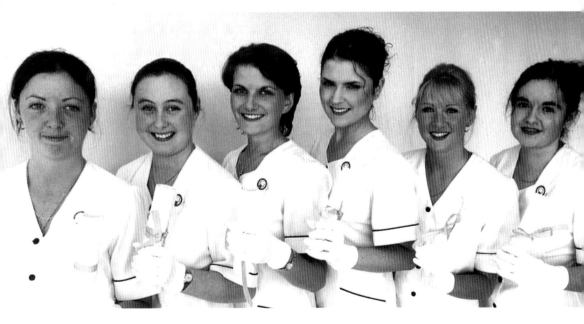

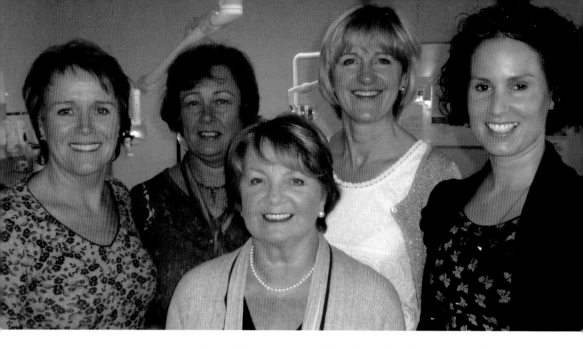

School of Dental Hygiene
tutors, 2013:
(left to right)
Clare Murphy,
Martina Collins,
Anne Houlihan,
Anne O'Keeffe,
Caroline Horgan.
COURTESY ANNE O'KEEFFE

a member of the part-time clinical staff in Restorative Dentistry for many years, and served as president of the Dental Council from 2005 to 2010). The two-year full-time programme features both classroom and clinical components undertaken at UCC and CUDSH. The qualification is recognised in Australia, Canada, the United States and elsewhere, subject to a registration-board exam. The annual student intake has increased from four to the current fourteen. Only one Cork dental hygienist graduate has been male (Neil Cullen, who qualified in 2003), though this is not inconsistent with international norms. A number of recent graduates have gone on to study dentistry.

The dental-nursing and dental-hygiene programmes have been success stories in Cork. They have adapted to changes in the field, and have developed a cadre of strong teachers, many of whom pursued higher degrees in teaching to improve their performance. Beyond the training provided to graduates, both programmes improved the school's clinical environment and BDS learning experience. At an institutional level they also altered the gender balance within CUDSH. Up until the 1970s, female BDS students were a minority and women teaching staff were rare. Now, women make up a majority of the school's students, and feature prominently in the institution's administration staff and faculty. This completed the modernisation of the Cork University Dental School and Hospital.

DENTAL TECHNICIANS

CUDSH staff has included a dental mechanic since its foundation. Responsible for constructing and repairing bridges, crowns, implants, dentures and orthodontic appliances, the dental mechanic is a critical member of the dental team. Until recently, the training for this career operated strictly on an apprenticeship system, though diploma courses have become increasingly common. Since the 1950s, the hospital has employed a new apprentice mechanic every five years. From 1983 to 1990, CUDSH ran four-year paid apprenticeships for dental technicians. The programme was sponsored by AnCO (the national training and employment agency; now FÁS). During their first three years, students received instruction at both CUDSH and Cork Regional Technical College (now Cork Institute of Technology). The fourth (final) year was comprised of on-the-job-training in a sponsored dental laboratory. Much of the teaching at CUDSH was provided by hospital technician Joe Hallissey, who remains one of the longest-tenured members of the school staff. Unfortunately, in 1990 AnCO discontinued the scheme. During its brief but successful operation, the apprenticeship programme produced a new generation of dental mechanics, who can still be found in dental laboratories across Ireland.

ORAL EPIDEMIOLOGY & THE ORAL HEALTH RESEARCH CENTRE

In 1965 CUDSH established the Special Studies in Dental Caries and Fluorides to monitor the effects of water fluoridation. In 1967 the special-unit director Chris Collins hired Denis O'Mullane to

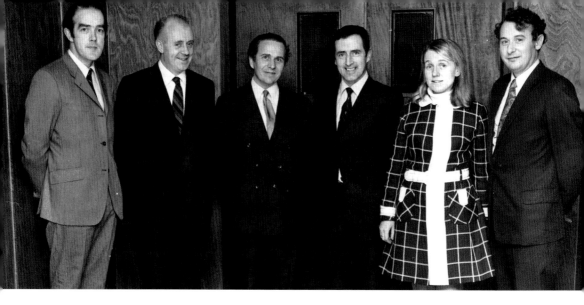

Foundation meeting of the Irish Society of Dentistry for Children, 1971: (left to right) V. Bluett, C. Collins, N. Swallow, D. O'Mullane, G. Lucey, T. Holland.

COURTESY: TIM HOLLAND

assist in, for example, monitoring the effects of water fluoridation (the Cork City Study) and in accessing the effectiveness of a fluoride mouth rinse (the Fermoy Fluoride Mouth Rinse Study).

At that time, the Special Studies on Dental Caries and Fluorides offices resided on the first floor of 4 St John's Terrace, a former residential home close to the North Infirmary purchased by CUDSH. From 1967 to 1972, its staff consisted of researchers Chris Collins and Denis O'Mullane, with Theresa O'Mahony, Yvonne Kelly and Mary Heffernan acting as recorders and fieldwork coordinators. Theresa O'Mahony registered for CUDSH's first course in dental nursing in 1969. Chris Collins left to commence private practice in Cork city. Denis O'Mullane departed for a lecturing position at the University of Manchester Dental School, which historically enjoyed close links with Cork. Dr Jim Mageean succeeded Chris Collins as head of the department and head of the Epidemiology Special Unit.

Following his six-year tenure in Manchester, Denis O'Mullane was appointed Ireland's Department of Health chief dental officer. He served in that position from 1978 to 1982, before returning to Cork as head of the Department of Preventive and Paediatric Dentistry. On his arrival, he installed a rigorous research regime that brought a number of high-profile projects to Cork.

At this stage, international dentistry recognised the need for ongoing research to determine the effectiveness and efficiency of dental-health services. On this basis, in 1984 the Oral Health Services Research Centre (OHSRC) was established in Cork to work with the Department of Health, various Health Boards, international bodies and private industry. The centre's first major initiative was the 1983 National Survey of Children's Dental Health, commissioned by the Department of Health. The study's principal investigator was Denis O'Mullane, and he hired as his research fellow Helen Whelton, who has been a member of the Oral Epidemiology Group in Cork University Dental School and Hospital since then. The centre's activities expanded during the late 1980s and early 1990s, through links with the EU, the Health Research Board and private industry, such as the companies Unilever and Proctor and Gamble. The OHSRC was initially sited

Examining a participant in the North Wales Schoolchildren Study, circa 1989. Courtesy CUDSH

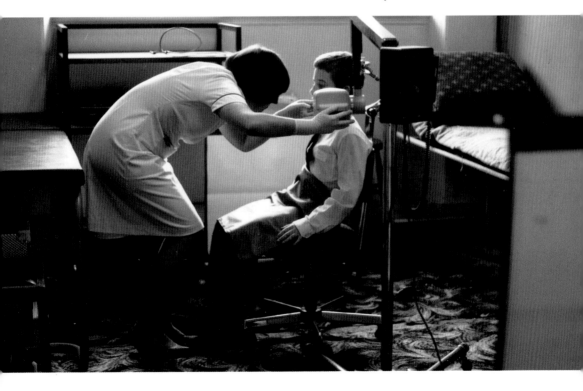

in the dental hospital in the offices of the Preventive and Paediatric Dentistry. The centre later moved to Askive House on Donovan's Road, and then for a number of years occupied the first floor of the Farm Centre at Dennehy's Cross.

In the early 1990s, the centre received a major research grant from Pfizer Corporation to study the effectiveness of a pre-brushing rinse. About the same time, the centre undertook a three-year study of toothpaste, underwritten by the Unilever Dental Research Group and involving 3,500 north Wales schoolchildren. These two commissioned studies marked a considerable expansion of the Oral Health Services Research Centre. They also necessitated a mobile unit kept in the dental-hospital car park. UCC saw the potential of the OHSRC, and approved the construction of its own home attached to the dental hospital. The university would not pay for the new building, so the OHSRC financed construction itself via a bank mortgage. That loan was paid off by allocating a fixed percentage of all OHSRC grants received from such funding bodies as the EU, the Department of Health, various Health Boards, the Health Research Board and the oral-health-care industry. Dr Helen Whelton and Kathryn Neville (chief administrator of the OHSRC) designed the new structure in consultation with architect Ger McCarthy.

In its new premises, the OHSRC has become an internationally recognised centre of excellence. It has built an extensive publication record in peer-reviewed journals, and has repeatedly secured funding from the EU. Numerous national oral-health surveys have been carried out, including National Adult Surveys in 1989/1990 and 2009, and a children's survey in 1984. It has also produced a national oral-health survey of adults with an intellectual disability, and a 2002 North/South children's survey covering both the Republic of Ireland and Northern Ireland. OHSRC has become critical in the training of postgraduate students, producing fourteen Ph.D.s and numerous masters degrees. The centre also established

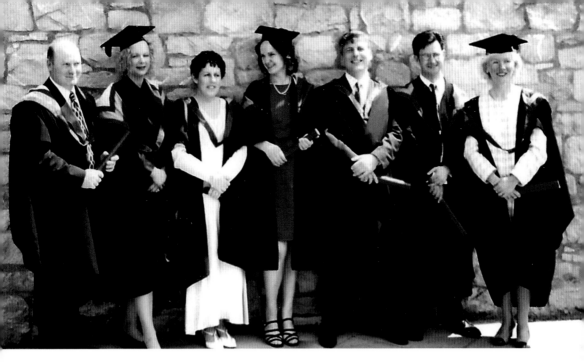

the successful Master in Dental Public Health (MDPH) degree, which takes in five to seven postgraduates every two years. Degree designer Helen Whelton succeeded Denis O'Mullane as OHSRC director following the latter's retirement in 2003. Since then, the OHSRC has conducted widely cited studies in the fields of fluorides and oral health, saliva and oral health, and epidemiological studies. A model of public and private educational collaboration, the OHSRC's international reputation can be seen in the recent election of Professor Whelton as president of the International Association for Dental Research. Recognition by international peers is perhaps the highest compliment an institution can receive. After receiving this honour, Professor Whelton has recently taken up the position of dean of the University of Leeds Dental School.

First graduating class, masters of public health, 1999: (left to right) Joe Green, Riana Clarke, Maura Haran, Helen Whelton, Michael Shanahan, Paul Beirne, Mary Ormbsy (née Boyce).
Courtesy Joe Green

6

A CENTURY OF TEACHING
& LEARNING, 1913–2013
----

*I*N July 1913 UCC President Bertram Windle established a four-year BDS-degree course. It would provide basic physical and biological-science courses (years one and two) on the UCC campus, and clinical aspects (years three and four) in a dental hospital operated by the North Charitable Infirmary.

Since that beginning, UCC's BDS-degree course maintained the division between basic science subjects offered on the UCC campus and the clinical component taught in the dental hospital. However, the degree also underwent major changes in its length, content and teaching methods. These adjustments accommodated a wider and continuous evolution in dental treatment, equipment, materials and safety guidelines.

FROM BLACKBOARD TO BLACKBOARD

In the early years, teachers used the 'chalk and talk' technique, outlining concepts on a blackboard with chalk. These were often illustrated with complex three-dimensional blackboard drawings, a skill perhaps best appreciated when considering the teaching of anatomy. In 2012 UCC's Glucksman Gallery marked the 1812 establishment of Ireland's first anatomy school (in Cork) with an exhibit showcasing elaborate coloured teaching diagrams by John Woodroofe and his fellow instructors. Their depictions of muscles, bones, arteries, veins, nerves and anatomical spaces were both educational and wonderful works of art. Over the years, UCC BDS students received instruction from similarly skilled teachers. For example, M.A. McConnell (professor of anatomy from the 1940s to the 1960s) usually entered the lecture theatre with his academic gown flowing and his hands armed with four different-coloured chalks. He would proceed to draw on the blackboard a three-dimensional illustration of the muscles of mastication and related blood and nerve supplies. At the end of the lecture, his technician Jim Raftery wiped everything from the blackboard. Such skills were not confined to anatomists, as lecturers in many subjects were often judged by both their eloquence and their chalk talent.

Many students found it an enormous challenge to take notes from lecturers whose pace varied widely. Some students could write lecture notes clearly, quickly and comprehensively, while simultaneously replicating blackboard diagrams legibly. Others plainly could not. This became apparent when students started their summer examination revisions (often signalled either by St Patrick's Day or the first cutting of the main-quad lawn). The discrepancy is now addressed in UCC's teaching and learning philosophy 'Multiple Intelligence', which acknowledges students' different learning styles and intelligence strengths (see below).

Blackboard and chalk served as the dominant teaching aids during the first half-century of Cork University Dental School and Hospital. During the 1960s, though, new teaching tools became more common. These included overhead and slide projectors, which used acetate sheets and photographed slides prepared before the lecture. Students also received (initially) mimeographed and (later) photocopied handouts to summarise lecture content and to explain assignments.

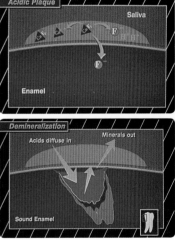

Teaching slides.
Courtesy CUDSH

As in other aspects of society, the development of computer technology dramatically impacted dental education. A major milestone was the creation of the PowerPoint presentation in 1987, an information technology that has improved since then. Perhaps the most significant computer teaching and learning aid is the electronic Blackboard, currently managed at UCC by Grace O'Leary. Under this system, a teacher may post their PowerPoint slide presentation on the UCC Blackboard some days before giving their lecture. Students can access and study the lecture prior to their teacher's presentation. They can also bring a hard copy to the lecture itself, and make their own notes on individual slides. After the lecture, the presentation can be stored by students on laptops and studied prior to examinations, and/or kept for future reference. This system embodies the multiple-intelligence philosophy, providing students with several methods for understanding what is being taught.

TEACHING & LEARNING

The Department of Education and Science in UCC enjoys an excellent international reputation for its work on the multiple intelligence (MI) concept, curriculum development and assessment methods. Founded in 2006 by Professor Áine Hyland, Ionad Bairre – UCC's Teaching and Learning Centre – has profoundly influenced teaching at the university. Research shows that multiple-intelligence teaching leads to greater involvement by students in their own instruction. Most of UCC's academic staff have adopted Teaching for Understanding (TFU) and Scholarship in Teaching and Learning (SoTL) concepts, which followed from the considerable efforts by Ionad Bairre faculty members Bettie Higgs and Marion McCarthy. The centre's Irish name is a translation of the UCC college-crest motto, 'Where Finbarr Taught let Munster Learn', which captures the dynamic synergy between teaching and learning at UCC.

CUDSH has embraced these education concepts. Many faculty members have completed teaching and learning certificates, diplomas or master degrees (see Appendix). Of special note are Dr Sharon Curtin and Dr Eleanor O'Sullivan, who have become known for instructing patients in smoking-cessation techniques. Dr Curtin is a behavioural scientist, the first to teach at a dental school in Ireland. Dr Mary McConnell has also undertaken notable work on visual-skills training and the use of art in learning. (A member of the part-time clinical staff in Restorative Dentistry, Dr McConnell is a noted artist and is married to Professor Robbie McConnell, the former head of CUDSH.) The teaching and training philosophy at CUDSH is to remain student-centred and patient-focused. Both students and patients seem to appreciate these emphases.

CHANGES IN THE UNDERGRADUATE DENTAL PROGRAMME OVER THE PAST CENTURY

The first four-year BDS-degree course announced in 1913 read as follows:

Course of Instruction for Degree of BDS
Approved by the National University of Ireland

First Year
Physics
Chemistry   *As First Year in Medicine*
Anatomy
First examination: chemistry and physics

....

Second Year
Anatomy and Practical Anatomy, Physiology and Histology, as in Medicine: but

(a) *In Anatomy – For the Dental Course in respect of the Central Nervous System the Abdomen and the Limbs, a less detailed knowledge will be required.*

(b) *In Physiology – For the Dental Course in respect of Physiology of the Central Nervous System, the Organs of Special Sense, Metabolism and the experimental Physiology of Muscle and Nerve, a less detailed knowledge will be required.*
General Hospital – Nine months

Second Examination : Anatomy and Physiology

....

Third Year
1) *Pathology. Lectures. One Term of Medicine Courses*
2) *Surgery. Lectures: the same as for Medicine Courses*
3) *Medicine. Lectures: the same as for Medicine Courses*
4) *Dental Surgery. One Term*
5) *Dental Mechanics. One Term*
6) *Dental Hospital. Six Months*

7) *Anaesthetics – as in Course in Surgery*
8) *Practical Pathology – as in Medicine Courses*
9) *Dental Hospital. Three Months*

Third Examination – Pathology and Practical Pathology
Surgery and Medicine

....

Fourth Year – Winter
1) *Dental Mechanics. One Term*
2) *Dental Surgery. One Term*
3) *Dental Hospital. Six Months*
4) *Orthodontia. One Term*
5) *Dental Materia Medica. One Term*

Final Examination for Degrees
1) *Dental Surgery and Pathology*
2) *Dental Mechanics*
3) *Operative Dentistry*
4) *Orthodontia*
5) *Dental Materia Medica*

The Examination must be passed in all five subjects at the same time.

Of the three subjects studied during the first year, only two, physics and chemistry, were examined. In the second year, the study of anatomy was continued (totalling two years) and examined. Course instruction required 'less detailed knowledge' of the central nervous system, abdomen and the limbs, but greater focus on the head and neck, which were more relevant to dentistry. A similar proviso emphasising oral biology was formulated for the physiology course. The second-year BDS examinations in anatomy and physiology featured questions on the subjects' general and dental aspects. Second-year students attended a general hospital for nine months, indicating a desire to align dentistry and medicine from the outset. Third-year studies blended general medical subjects (pathology, surgery, medicine and anaesthetics) and dental surgery and dental

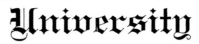

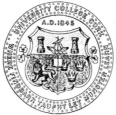

OFFICIAL GAZETTE.

Published under the Authority of the Governing Body.

Vol. iii.—No. 9.   TRINITY.   July, 1913.

CONTENTS.

liv.   DENTAL DEGREES AND DIPLOMAS.

It is comparatively but a few years ago since the Dental Act constituted persons practising that branch of medicine into a distinct profession, and it is only now that medical men and dentists are beginning to understand the full importance of that fact in relation to the now, but only now known, bearing of diseases of the teeth upon the general health of the body. Up to the present there has been no complete provision for the teaching of this important branch of medicine in Cork, and that largely because Cork, almost alone among the great cities of the three kingdoms, has been unprovided with any proper Dental Hospital or Dental Department at a General Hospital. It is true that there are dental surgeons of ability attached to several Cork Hospitals, but up to the present no provision has been made for any other treatment of the teeth than that of extraction. Now, as everyone knows, the extraction of the teeth nowadays is but a small part of the treatment available for the dentist. Conservative Dentistry, so called, has made enormous strides since the dental profession was properly constituted. There has, however, been no provision made to enable the poorer classes in Cork to profit by such treatment, though it was and is available for those who can afford to pay the ordinary fees of the qualified dental surgeon. That this was in no way the fault or desire of the dental practitioners is shown by the readiness with which they welcomed the suggestion of a Dental Hospital and placed their services fully, freely, and gratuitously at its disposal, to their great credit.

mechanics. A total of nine months' practical training in the dental hospital were also required. During their fourth (final) year, students treated patients at the dental hospital under supervision for nine months, while also studying theoretical aspects of dental mechanics, dental surgery, orthodontia and dental materia medica. To qualify for the degree, students were required to pass two fourth-year (final-year) examinations covering five subjects. These exam papers were entitled 'dental surgery' and 'mechanical dentistry'.

DYMPNA KAVANAGH:
CHIEF DENTAL OFFICER

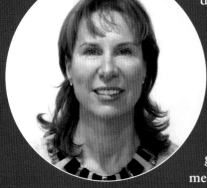

Dympna Kavanagh.

One of the school's most accomplished graduates of recent years is Dympna Kavanagh, Ireland's current chief dental officer. She is an exemplar of the school's proud tradition of public-health service.

While in secondary school in Tipperary town, Dr Kavanagh became interested in dentistry after spending a day with the local public-health dentist, the late Niamh O'Grady. 'She was an inspirational figure', Dympna recalled. 'I had always been into crafts and generally working with my hands and she inspired me to go for dentistry. I changed my application at the last minute and went to Cork Dental School.'

After obtaining a first-class-honours degree from Cork in 1987, Dympna moved to the UK to work in the National Health Service. While based at Guy's Hospital (King's College), she obtained an impressive array of academic certificates and diplomas. Throughout her career she has continued her education, while ensuring it was relevant to her day-to-day working life.

Dympna renewed her Cork connection by joining the Oral Health Services Research Centre as a researcher. While working, she undertook her Ph.D. thesis, 'Predicting High Caries Risk in Adolescents', and was awarded a Ph.D. in preventive and paediatric dentistry in 1994. She progressed through a series of public-health posts in the UK, and then in Ireland after returning home for good in 2001.

Currently, Dympna enjoys the distinction of serving in Irish dentistry's two most senior leadership posts. In 2010 the HSE named her 'oral health lead', responsible for planning, monitoring and evaluating public-dental-care services. Three years later, in 2013, the minister for health appointed Dr Kavanagh to the post of chief dental officer, Department of Health. In that role Dympna advises the Department of Health on all matters relating to oral health. Facing a challenging economic climate, she seeks to coordinate what she calls 'all the pieces of the jigsaw in Irish public dentistry'. During her upcoming tenure, Dympna intends to address crucial issues sooner rather than later. Aware of the progress achieved by her predecessors, she will also lay out a clear vision of the future for Irish dentistry.

Dympna has always sought to achieve a balance between her work and lifestyle. She, her husband (and former classmate) Joe Callanan (BDS 1987) and their two sons currently live in a restored Georgian house in Limerick city centre. Joe holds an offshore yachtmaster's certificate, and often sails in west Cork and France. When not promoting dental health, Dympna's favourite place is aboard a sailboat with her family. There she prefers to remain 'strictly crew'.

Over the next fifty years, adjustments were made to the BDS-degree programme, though the structure and subject content remained largely the same. A major change occurred in the 1940s when dental students were required to spend five years in university, adding one year to the degree programme. A new first year was designated 'pre-dental' and devoted to the study of physics, chemistry, botany and zoology. Initially, the pre-dental year also included instruction in sociology, psychology and philosophy. By 1963 these 'arts' subjects were reduced to an introductory philosophy course taught by the well-known Capuchin friar, Professor Peter Dempsey. The addition of the pre-dental year reflected the poor state of Irish secondary education at that time, since many schools did not have the teaching staff or laboratory facilities required to teach physics, chemistry or biology.

ASSESSMENT

During CUDSH's first half-century, student competency was assessed primarily through written examinations held at the end of the academic year. Questions from the final-year BDS written examinations over the years illustrate many changes in dental education and within the profession itself.

The first final-year BDS papers were set in 1915 and passed by students William Foley and Eugene Whelan. The two examination papers, dental surgery and mechanical dentistry, covered a total of five subjects. Dental-surgery questions focused primarily on complications arising from teeth extraction and dental and oral pathology ('How does arsenic devitalise a tooth?' 'What precautions must be taken when using it for this purpose?'). Mechanical-dentistry questions were directed towards the construction of dentures and splints, and the use and risks of soldering for these purposes. Materials mentioned were gold, vulcanite, bell metal, gun metal, babbitt metal and bronze ('Describe fully the process of vulcanisation of rubber.').

Orthodontics was covered even at this early stage of dentistry ('What are the advantages and disadvantages of fixed and removable apparatus in the treatment of irregularities?').

By 1920 the first questions appeared on restorative dentistry ('If a mandrel breaks in a root canal, what steps would you take for its removal? If you are unsuccessful in your efforts, what is the prognosis?'). Prevention also premiered as an exam topic ('How does saliva act (a) in preventing dental caries (b) on food stuffs which indirectly predispose to caries?'). Mechanical-dentistry papers focused primarily on materials used at that time, especially gold, silver and porcelain. One question, however, indicated more-advanced restorative restorations ('What are the advantages and disadvantages of (a) a cast gold inlay (b) a banded crown (c) an all porcelain crown?').

In 1925 the first question in periodontology appeared ('Classify the varieties of stomatitis and how to treat any one form of same.'). The state of local anaesthetics was reflected in a 1935 question ('Why is novocaine used as an anaesthetic in preference to cocaine? What kind of solution would you use to dissolve the drug and what is the maximum safe dose?'). The 1936 dental-surgery BDS paper shows different aesthetic treatments proscribed for men and women ('Describe the best method of restoration of caries on the buccal side of a central incisor in a young woman. Describe the technique.').

The year 1945 saw the first queries on the properties of silver/tin amalgams ('Give an account of the factors which affect the setting and properties of silver/tin amalgams.'). The same year's exam reflected the widespread use of nitrous oxide and chloroform as general anaesthetics in dental practice ('Describe the appearance of the pupils in the first and third stages of chloroform anaesthesia and the third stage of nitrous oxide anaesthesia.'). By 1949 questions were addressing more-complex restorative dentistry ('Describe the preparation and restoration of an MOD cavity.').

The 1950 exam mentioned penicillin for the first time ('What pharmacological considerations would enable you to decide as between penicillin and sulphatriad in a case of sepsis?'). Jacket-crown preparation showed up initially in 1955 ('Describe the operative procedures for the preparation of an acrylic jacket crown.'). Though periodic orthodontic questions had appeared previously, 1955 marked the first full paper devoted to orthodontics, and followed the appointment of Professor Rodney Dockrell from the Dublin dental school as a visiting part-time professor in orthodontics. Alginates arrived with the 1960 exam in dental prosthetics ('Compare plaster-of-Paris and the alginates as impression materials for edentulous cases.').

As the school entered its second half-century, questions on periodontal conditions became more specific, as seen in the 1965 BDS paper ('What are the causes, signs and symptoms of acute local periodontitis? Discuss its treatment.'). Dental-prosthetics questions still related almost exclusively to the construction of full upper, lower and partial dentures. Following the 1965 appointment of Chris Collins as statutory lecturer in preventive dentistry, the first BDS paper in preventive dentistry appeared. In 1970 dental public health made its exam premier ('Discuss the role of dental surveys in public health dentistry.'). The extraction of permanent incisors to improve the appearance of a young adult (rather than orthodontic treatment) appeared in a 1970 question ('An 18-year-old patient who has an angle class II division/malocclusion requests that her four upper incisor teeth are extracted and that an immediate replacement denture is constructed to markedly improve her appearance. Discuss the problems associated with such a request in order that the patient understands the treatment required.').

The 1980 exam saw the first reference to glass ionomer ('Write a short note on "Glass Ionomer cements".'). By 1985 the use of resin-bonded cast-metal restorations had appeared ('Discuss the history, development and use of resin-bonded cast-metal bridgework.'). A question in 1990 showed the common usage of composite materials ('Compare the properties of amalgam and composites as a posterior filling material.').

The improvements in Irish oral health over time were considered in the 1996 preventive and paediatric BDS paper ('Describe the recent improvement in the oral health of children and adults in the Republic of Ireland. Give reasons for these improvements.'). By 2000 the routine provision of primary care for patients with disabilities was seen in the preventive and paediatric dentistry paper ('Briefly outline the dental management of children with the following: (a.) Congenital heart disease (b.) Haemophilia (c.) A history of radiotherapy to the head and neck.'). Students also had to consider dental trauma in children ('Describe your management of an avulsed permanent incisor in a child, with particular reference to the immediate and long-term consequences of this injury.').

The decline in adult tooth loss and the shift to preservation of natural teeth in the elderly led to an increase of gerodontology questions asked in 2003 ('Discuss the problems that may be encountered when providing restorative dental care for elderly patients.'). Widespread use of bonding agents in restorative treatment was apparent in a 2007 question ('Discuss the role of adhesive restorative materials in clinical dentistry.'). The 2009 restorative BDS paper reflected profound changes in prosthetic dentistry during recent decades ('Removable partial dentures are a thing of the past. Discuss this statement.'). Perhaps a less welcomed aspect of contemporary dentistry can be seen in the 2010 question that considers the legal consequences of patient care ('When instrumenting a lower incisor an endodontic file fractures in the apical third of the canal. Discuss your management of this case from both a legal and a clinical standpoint.').

CHANGES TO THE BDS PROGRAMME

The school's appointment in 1965 of three full-time professors – in restorative dentistry (Brian Barrett), oral surgery (Gordon Russell) and orthodontics (Mary Hegarty) – ushered in a new era. They were followed by a new chair in prosthetics (Bill McCullough, appointed in 1969) and the appointment of Chris Collins as head of preventive and paediatric dentistry. At this time, school officials came to recognise the necessity of a five-year course for the BDS degree to develop the competencies, knowledge and professional attitudes required to practise dentistry. Students had previously acquired competency in the basic sciences during the pre-dental year. Now, that knowledge was covered by stricter university-entry requirements, which included high marks in the Leaving Certificate for such subjects as chemistry, physics and biology.

After Ireland joined the European Union (EU) in 1973 (then called the European Economic Community (EEC)), CUDSH adhered to EEC/EU education directives. One such directive, 78/686/EEC, ratified in 1978, called on member states to mutually recognise dental degrees adhering to basic standards. Essentially, this directive (together with further amendments over the next thirty-five years) led to the current standard of a five-year BDS undergraduate programme in EU member states. The same year, directive 78/687/EEC recognised orthodontics and oral surgery as specialities within the EEC. To facilitate the implementation of these directives in Ireland, an EEC (later EU) Dental Liaison Committee was established. UCC graduate Joe Lemasney (BDS 1957) served on this committee for many years, and was subsequently elected its chairman. Indicative of Cork's dental familial network, Joe married his classmate Eithne Twomey (BDS 1957), and the couple sent two children to CUDSH, Barry (BDS 1982) and Niall (BDS 1983).

Developments within the EU led to discussions in Ireland about the state of the profession by dental professionals, members

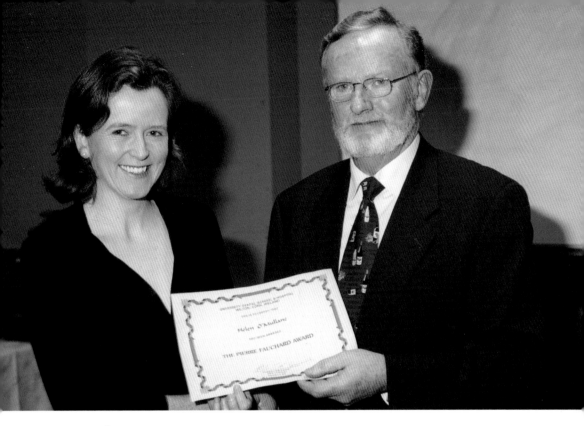

of Dáil Éireann and the Department of Health. These culminated in the passage of the new Dentists Act, 1985. It replaced the 1928 Dentists Act, and established a Dental Council to replace the old Dental Board. Professors Brian Barrett and Denis O'Mullane represented UCC on the first council, with the latter serving as chairman of the Auxiliary Dental Workers' Committee. That body ultimately facilitated the establishment of the grade of dental hygienist as a recognised member of the dental team in Ireland (see Chapter 5).

Another Irish educational milestone was the 1978 introduction of the CAO (Central Applications Office) points system for students applying for university courses. To study for a BDS degree, new students needed satisfactory Leaving Certificate marks in the basic science subjects. In 2013, for example, the relevant minimum requirement was a mark of 'HC3 in chemistry and either physics or biology and passes at H or C level in Leaving Cert for Irish, English and another language and mathematics'.

2001 Pierre Fauchard Award presented to Helen O'Mullane by UCC president, Gerry Wrixon.

Courtesy Denis O'Mullane

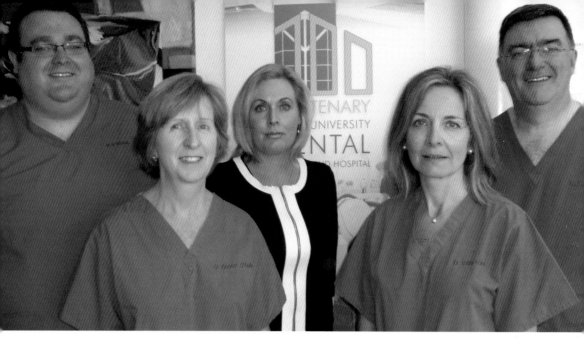

BDS course coordinators, 2013: (left to right) G. McKenna (4th year), E. O'Sullivan (1st year), S. Curtin (2nd year), E. Allen (3rd year), F. Burke (5th (final) year).
COURTESY NEIL NASH

Long-term changes in the undergraduate BDS programme can be seen by studying the current (2012–13) UCC Calendar, Book of Modules, and Marks and Standards. These outline the five-year BDS-degree's entry requirements, course structure, covered subjects and assessment procedures for each subject area.

The current subject areas resemble those studied from 1913 to 1963, though the programme structure has undergone major changes. The degree now practises vertical integration of clinical subjects from first year onwards (for example, during every year of study, students receive instruction on behavioural sciences and ethics). In the early 1980s, CUDSH moved to a modular and associated credit system. In each year, subject areas consist of modules measured by credits. A module may consist of 5, 10, 15 or 20 credits. For each of the five years, students must pass modules totalling 60 credits, giving a total value of 300 credits for the BDS degree.

First-year features modules in anatomy, physiology and biochemistry. It also includes a course in 'fundamentals of dental practice', worth 20 credits of the year's total of 60. This module covers a wide range of topics, such as the role of behavioural sciences in clinical dentistry. Its assessment procedures typifies the trend towards more innovative examination techniques, with half of the marks awarded by continuous assessment and half by oral assessment. The module co-coordinator is Dr Eleanor O'Sullivan, who coordinates the entire first-year programme.

The second-year course (co-coordinator Dr Sharon Curtin) again illustrates the move towards vertical integration. Ten credits (of 60) are devoted to an introductory course in restorative dentistry, which includes diverse topics such as communication skills, smoking-cessation protocols and infection control.

The third-year course (co-coordinator Dr Edith Allen) offers three modules on restorative dentistry, worth 45 credits. Students learn to take a patient's history, examine and diagnose common dental diseases, give local anaesthesia, provide preventive care, and manage mild periodontal conditions. They also develop communication skills and relaxation techniques for anxious patients.

The fourth-year course (co-coordinator Dr Gerry McKenna) and fifth- (final) year course (co-coordinator Dr Frank Burke) are entirely devoted to the following clinical-dental subject areas:

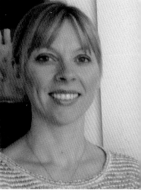

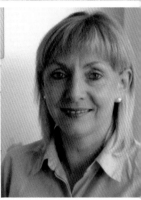

- Restorative dentistry (head, Professor Finbarr Allen), including periodontology and adult oral health;
- Oral health and development (head, Professor Martin Kinirons), including orthodontics, paediatric dentistry, preventive dentistry and dental public health;
- Dental surgery (head, Professor Duncan Sleeman), including oral surgery, oral medicine, oral pathology and oral radiology.

Dental nursing tutors Siobhán Shakeshaft (top) and Mary Harrington.
COURTESY NEIL NASH

Clinical skills (treating patients) are taught in the dental hospital under supervision in dental clinics, in which there are a total of eighty dental chairs. Students are continuously assessed by the allocation of a grade for each procedure completed during the two years of the course. These marks are aggregated and contribute to the final BDS examination score.

Another feature of the BDS undergraduate degree programme

is worth noting. A B.Sc. (ordinary) degree in oral-health studies has been created for the small number of students who pass their third-year dental exams but choose to no longer study dentistry.

CHANGES IN ASSESSMENT TECHNIQUES

BDS-degree graduates should possess the competencies, knowledge and skills needed to register with the Dental Council of Ireland. This qualification allows freedom of movement within the EU and the right of establishment for EU citizens in member states.

Each module is assessed separately, according to its own requirements. While student assessment used to be based primarily on examinations, continuous assessment has become more common in recent years. This trend better accommodates the diverse theoretical, clinical, manual-dexterity, and social and problem-solving skills needed upon completion of the BDS degree. Assessment techniques include essay-type examinations, literature reviews, competency tests, clinical examinations, electronic portfolios of reflective practice, and traditional written examinations. Many elements of the BDS degree now carry marks forward from year to year. For example, accumulated marks currently make up over half of the final-year exam results in restorative dentistry.

CHANGES IN PRACTICES OF DENTISTRY, 1913–2013: FROM THE VERTICAL TO THE HORIZONTAL

This book's cover photograph shows Cork graduate Willie Palmer (BDS 1948) treating a patient in Spa National School outside Tralee circa 1955. The patient is sitting upright and the dentist is standing up and using a foot drill. This patient and dentist position was the norm during CUDSH's first half-century. Two of this book's authors – Denis O'Mullane (BDS 1960) and Tim Holland

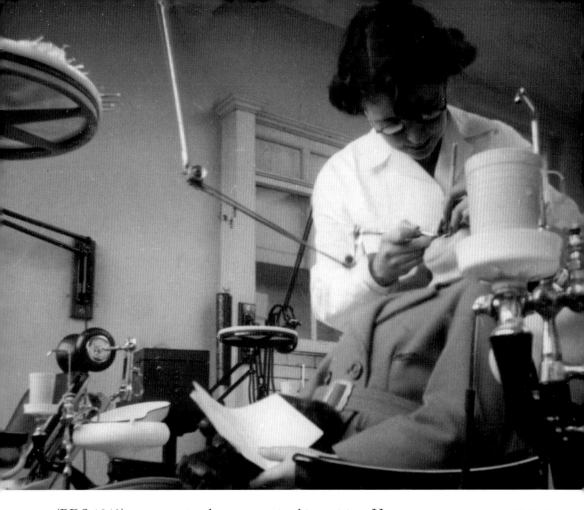

(BDS 1963) – were trained to operate in this position. However, scientific literature during the 1960s reported high levels of musculoskeletal ailments amongst dentists, including headaches and lower back pain. This resulted in ergonomic consideration in the design of dental surgeries and dental equipment (especially stools and chairs). Many dentists who practised in the late Sixties and early Seventies remember the introduction of the 'Murray stool'. The wheeled stool allowed the dentist to sit and move around the dental chair, treating a patient without standing. At the same time, electrically powered dental chairs became more sophisticated, allowing the dentist to raise and lower the patient's seat and chair back. This led to the universal adoption of the patient lying in the prone position, and the dentist and dental nurse sitting at the

Student dentist Sheila Ahern treating patient in standing position, circa 1955.
Courtesy Ger Fitzgerald

PETER CUDMORE: CLINICAL TEACHER

Paediatric dentistry has been well served by Peter Cudmore (BDS 1974), one of the department's most popular staff members during nearly forty years of service.

A Cork native educated at Glenstal Abbey, Peter was initially drawn to dentistry because he loved science and worked well with his hands. After qualifying, he followed his colleagues into private practice in England. Returning home a year later, Peter established his own practice in Cork city, but first had to wait for the arrival of his office equipment from his supplier. At a loose end, he accepted a four-month full-time house-surgeon position at CUDSH. The experience was a revelation, providing him with his 'best four months of dentistry'. For the first time, Peter looked forward to going into work after a weekend. While he developed his private practice, Peter accepted sessional clinical work at the hospital to fill any gaps in his schedule. Though his practice improved, Peter still continued to teach at the hospital, to the dismay of his accountant. Normally working on his own, Peter valued the social aspect of the dental hospital, where he could confer with top experts in the field and compare notes with fellow dentists in practice. The business side of practice management never attracted him, and he felt unburdened by such concerns at the hospital. There, he found pure dentistry combined with a collegial atmosphere and the challenge of managing both patients and students.

Peter Cudmore.

Without any particular design, Peter gravitated towards paediatric dentistry, treating children between the ages of six and twelve. He considered this a difficult teaching area, as some students developed a fear of treating children. Students could find it difficult to establish a rapport with the child, or could not deal with multiple distractions, or grew terrified of making a mistake on a vulnerable patient in front of their mother or father. Many students mistakenly communicated with the parent instead of the patient, or aroused the child's disgust by speaking to them in baby talk. Sometimes, the child sensed the unease of the student practitioner and became unruly. As he described it, Peter was required 'to train a nervous student to treat a nervous mother and child'. He impressed students with an easy bedside manner and calmness during emergencies. Like most clinical-staff members, he also imparted professional wisdom not always found in textbooks, accessing his own experience in private practice. In this way, the part-time staff carried on some of the best features of the old dental-apprenticeship system.

Peter Cudmore has become a highly respected member of the clinical-teaching staff during one of the longest tenures in CUDSH history. From that perspective, it is interesting to note that he missed the intimacy of the old dental hospital. Despite the poor facilities, it mandated close personal interaction with one's peers, which encouraged institutional loyalty and comradeship. While the new hospital facilities are eminently superior, he considers its departmentalisation less social than the old home on John Redmond Street.

Peter sold his private practice in 2005, but has remained two days a week at the dental hospital. He frequently recuperates from his interactions with nervous parents and nervous students by sailing off the south coast of Ireland.

side of the patient's head (see photo on back cover). The dentist and nurse's backs remain upright, with their femurs parallel to the floor. The patient's oral cavity is situated so that it can be accessed without the dentist or nurse crouching. Modern dental surgeries (including equipment, stools, chairs, instruments and materials) are designed to minimise physical and mental stress. Dentists, dental nurses and dental hygienists are now taught to ensure that ergonomically sound working positions are established from the outset, practised routinely, and maintained throughout their working life.

FOOT POWER TO ELECTRIC POWER

Extraction of teeth and their replacement with dentures was the most common treatment option offered in the early years of CUDSH. Conservative dentistry (mainly fillings, crowns or inlays) was also taught from the outset. These approaches inevitably required the drilling of enamel, which is the body's hardest tissue. Increased efficiency in drilling of human teeth challenged dental researchers throughout the past century. From 1913 to 1932, Cork dental students used a foot-powered drill to prepare a tooth for restoration. The dentist generated the machine power by using a pedal motion similar to that used in spinning wheels at the time. It has been reported that in this period, dentists with extensive conservative practices could be recognised by the increased size of their 'pedal leg' and occasionally by a pronounced limp. In the same era, a hand-operated 'chip syringe' provided the air blast required to rid the cavity of accumulated saliva during preparation (the instrument was a rubber ball with a metal air duct). Two Ritter electric dental engines and electric air syringes were installed in the Cork dental hospital during 1932, though foot drills continued in Irish dental practices and the school dental service until the 1950s. The rotation speed of the cutting 'bur' on the hand piece continued to be relatively slow. This made the cutting and shaping of enamel difficult for the dentist and uncomfortable for the patient. The major breakthrough in tooth-cutting technology came with the air rotor, which was introduced into the Cork dental hospital in 1963. It made the cutting of tooth tissue easier, quicker and more comfortable for the patient. Over the last fifty years, the technology for preparing tooth tissue for restoration has become increasingly sophisticated. Neither dentists nor patients miss the long drilling time previously required.

INFECTION CONTROL/HEALTH & SAFETY/ RADIATION PROTECTION

Safety guidelines to protect patients and staff have been updated regularly over the years. Senior members of the dental profession will recall boiling a single local anaesthetic needle to be used again and again on different patients. Sterilisation at that time meant placing instruments in boiling water after use on the patient, and reusing them after twenty or thirty minutes at boiling point. The introduction of the autoclave (pressurised steam) marked the beginning of the current system of sterilisation of instruments in places such as the Cork dental hospital. Instrument and equip-ment sterilisation at CUDSH is now rigorous, highly technical and scientifically based. During the tenure of Professor Robbie McConnell as head of school and Kathryn Neville as manager, the hospital installed a state-of-the-art Central Sterile Services Department (CSSD) to sterilise all instruments centrally. Instruments are now classified according to their risk of transmit-ting infection. For example, they may be prioritised by whether they penetrated tissue, touched the oral mucosa, or only came into to contact with skin (such as a hose on an X-ray head). Currently run by Mary Moloney, the CSSD has four separate areas: cleaning, disinfection, sterilisation and storage. Regulations require that each instrument's sterilisation history is fully recorded and traceable.

That record is placed in the patient's notes, making it available in the event of any patient, student or dentist developing an infection. By using these techniques, students familiarise themselves with the principles and procedures of infection control, which they will use from the start of their professional careers.

Cross-infection control can be seen in the way clinicians dress at CUDSH. Clinicians now wear disposable surgical gloves and masks, and the clinical staff and students change into surgical gowns when entering clinical areas of the dental hospital. Gowns are not worn outside of the hospital. The patient and dentist also wear protective glasses. The posed photograph on the back cover of this book illustrates the ergonomically correct operating positions. The attire of the patient (Kate McSweeney), dentist (Dr Joe McKenna), student (Sorcha Harding) and dental nurse (Amelia Spillane) meet health-and-safety infection-control protocols, and is a stark comparison with the photograph on the book's front cover.

Precautions to protect the operators and patients from excessive radiation are now well established. While students are taught the diagnostic value of radiography, they are strongly discouraged from taking 'routine' X-rays. Patients are X-rayed only when there is reason to believe the radiograph will help in a diagnosis and the formulation of a treatment plan.

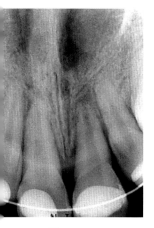

X-ray. Courtesy CUDSH

Two of this book's co-authors were trained with a number of now-obsolete instruments and treatment methods. Sometimes, they shudder at memories of reused needles, agonisingly slow drilling into a cavity, or the wearing of clinical clothes in unsanitary environments. However, when the history is written of the Cork University Dental School and Hospital's second century, one can be certain that some of today's practices will be considered arcane and bewildering. A major theme of this historical narrative has been the continued evolution of dental education and dentistry carried out by professionals dedicated to their craft. There is little to doubt that leaps in knowledge and technique will continue in coming decades.

7

THE DENTAL-SCHOOL COMMUNITY

*T*HE Cork University Dental School and Hospital is more than just a physical space. It is a community comprised of students, teachers, staff and graduates, bound together by common interests and experiences. Every autumn for the past century, an incoming class of first-year dental students joins that community.

Like all university students, Cork dental graduates retain fond memories of happy times and daring deeds at college. A few safe generalisations can be made about a century of undergraduate days. Students today dance less than their predecessors. Earlier generations of students had little pocket money, no cars and remained in Cork at weekends. The sexual revolution of the 1970s altered social expectations, and today's students are much more diverse in terms of race, religion and attitudes towards sexuality. Yet some common themes run through the decades: dental students sought entertainment during spare time, they developed close friendships with classmates, and they periodically blew off steam.

CONNECTIONS

In conversations with CUDSH graduates, nearly all referred to lifelong friendships established during their undergraduate progression. Most alumni remain in close contact with some classmates, and many are familiar with comings and goings of an expansive network of former colleagues. This bond can be attributed in part to the considerable time students spent together, often in close proximity and sometimes under trying circumstances. Not surprisingly, such intimacy produced romances, and in many cases led to marriages between dental students, as well as with dental nurses and dental hygienists. In the late 1950s, for example, nearly forty per cent of women graduates married another dentist from the school, though this trend eventually tapered off.

Reflecting the student *esprit de corps* was the Cork Dental Student Society, which contributed so much to saving the school.

One of its key leaders, Dan Finn, later recalled the strong links among his classmates, who remain close to this day. Though difficult to quantify, there seems a likely correlation between student activism and class camaraderie. Cross-border collegiality also featured in Cork students' involvement in the Irish Dental Students' Association, established in 1970. Cork students fondly recalled their Northern Ireland counterparts from Queen's University Belfast dental school, who had a reputation as 'a wild bunch' at the annual association congress. North–South relations within this body seemed to have been largely unaffected by the Northern Ireland Troubles. Like the experience of dental emigrants to Britain, it seems that professionalism frequently trumped nationalism, even during times of traumatic political strife.

SOCIALISING

The current Irish undergraduate drinking culture appears to be a relatively recent innovation. Earlier students typically usually possessed only enough pocket money to subsidise moderate drinking, while women faced a social taboo when entering a pub. Up until the late 1960s, students on campus practised self-segregation by patronising the gendered 'Men's Club' (now called 'The Old Bar') and the 'Ladies' Club' (now part of the staff restaurant). The former premises included a pool table and could accommodate numerous undergraduates, while the latter had poorer facilities, which reflected women's subordinate status at UCC. Card playing and other games featured prominently in both locales. Many students drank socially but not necessarily to excess, and it was quite normal for classmates to spend hours in the pub nursing non-alcoholic drinks.

During the past hundred years, a few pubs stand out. During the school's first half-century, the pre-eminent establishment was Pat Buckley's bar, at 14 John Redmond Street, just across the road

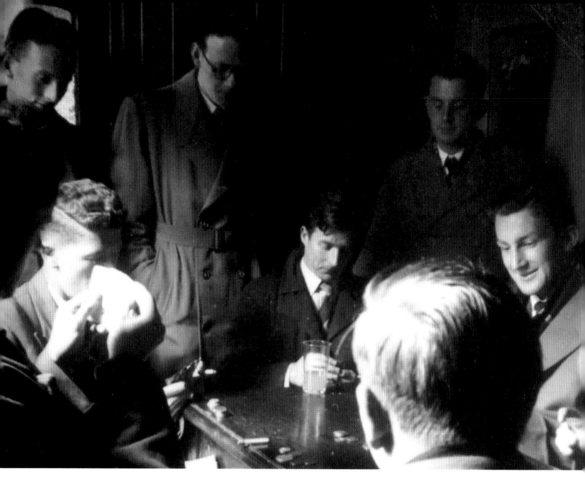

Dental students in Buckley's pub, circa 1955.
Courtesy Ger Fitzgerald

from the dental hospital. Run with great efficiency by Ms Buckley, it was very much a public house, though more like a sitting room than a modern bar. Ms Buckley allowed students to run tabs kept neatly on a slate behind the counter. Trusted students maintained their own tally and even drew pints themselves when Ms Buckley was unavailable, dutifully adding them to their tab. In turn, Ms Buckley usually notified her charges if she received a telephone call from the dental hospital looking for a wayward student. When some of those graduates moved to England to work, they provided a remittance to Ms Buckley, paying off their bar bill with their first pay cheques.

Students in the 1970s migrated down the lane to Pa Johnson's on Devonshire Street, one of the most beloved pubs in the city. Tiny and crammed with characters, it was renowned for its piano and close association with Irish showbands. The head barman, Barry Johnson (Pa's son), befriended numerous dental students roughly his own age. Barry essentially became an associate member of the CUDSH student body, attending social events and developing a number of lifelong dental friendships. The student connection to Pa Johnson's broke when the dental hospital moved to its new location in Wilton. Regardless, Barry Johnson came away satisfied, as he married Mary McCarthy, a nurse in the dental hospital. Pa Johnson's nearly fell victim to the Celtic Tiger building craze when the old premises was purchased for a housing block and completely demolished. However, it has been reincarnated in a new structure, and its piano can still be heard on John Redmond Street.

Since moving to Wilton, dental students have less immediate access to Cork's finer drinking establishments. There is no longer a designated student pub, though students and staff can often be sighted in the Bishopstown Bar or tackling a carvery meal at the Wilton Pub and Restaurant. More often, students associate in smaller groups in the city centre. Indeed, the diminished social dimension is a downside to the dental hospital's move from the city centre.

ACTIVITIES

CUDSH graduates generally agree that undergraduates possessed less spending money before the late 1990s. At a time of high Irish unemployment, students commonly took summer jobs in London to make cash for the upcoming term. Popular employers were London Transport, British Rail and Wall's ice-cream factory. Wall's paid students double-time for working in the giant freezer, a bonus offset by chattering teeth and frozen extremities. Among the undergrads employed by British Rail, two stories are sometimes told by graduates. One dental student (and future faculty member) worked as a porter at St Pancras railway station. Asked by an elderly gentleman if the soon-to-depart train at the platform was the 10 pm train to Watford (a thirty-minute journey), the student replied authoritatively that it was. Unfortunately, only after the train pulled away did the student realise that the gentleman had in fact boarded the non-stop overnight express to Glasgow. Another student porter at Paddington station had just failed his first-year biochemistry exam, externed by the Nobel Prize-winning chemist, Sir Hans Krebs. By happy coincidence, Dr Krebs stepped onto the student's platform dragging an enormous trunk. The student apparently had the pleasure of telling the bewildered Dr Krebs, 'you can carry your own bloody bags'.

Before the 1970s, students dressed more formally, with skirts usually worn by women and jackets and ties by men. Up until the late 1950s, black gowns were required when attending lectures at UCC; a common classroom prank was cutting a hole in the back of the gown of a student seated in front. Students had to cross town from their clinical work at the dental hospital to academic lectures on the UCC campus, and it was not unusual to see one bicycle with three gowned students on board, heading to UCC at speed. One garda who wore white gloves and theatrically directed traffic at the junction of Patrick Street and Camden Quay took special satisfaction in reprimanding student bicycle transgressors.

Writing in 1982, Cork dental-school historian Ray Gamble (a graduate and long-time member of staff) noted how the cross-town trip affected student attendance:

> Latter day students may be interested to learn that lack of punctuality was frowned upon. One such occurrence was sufficient to put the student before the Dean. Those familiar with the topography of Cork and its Venetian-like channels spanned in former days by lifting and lateral swing-opening bridges will appreciate the oft used excuse, 'The bridge was up, sir', soon lost its efficacy. The advent

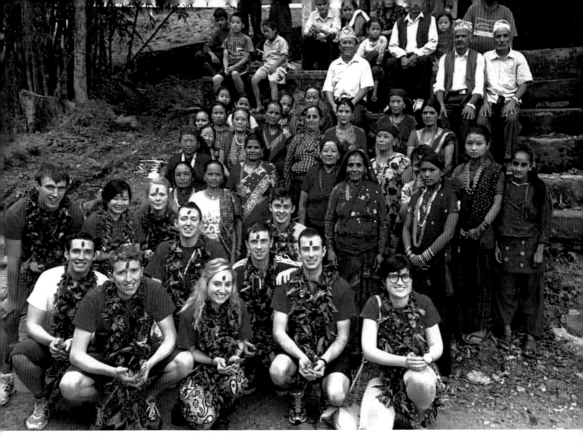

Fourth-year dental students in Taksar, Napal, 2013: (back, left to right) I. Murphy, S. Goh, L. Clifford; (centre, left to right) C. O'Meara, R. Fitzgerald, C. Carroll, T. Horgan; (front, left to right) P. Hennessy, P. Sinnott, J. Donovan, L. Rawle. At the back (centre) is village president, Tek Bahadur Gurung.

COURTESY JOEY DONOVAN

of deeper draft ships and the closing of the Cork quays by fixed pontics, has deprived absentees of a plausible tale.

One consistent feature of dental-student life was the close friendship that developed between students and the part-time clinical staff. Invariably, they were great allies of the students, who often recall stories of staff encouragement during clinical and theoretical training. Such generosity disappeared at the annual staff-versus-students soccer match, which was one of the year's big social occasions. Close bonds also developed with the nurses, secretaries and technicians. Often feeling great pressure at exam time, students frequently confided in the staff, who usually offered a helping hand or sympathetic ear. Bríd Ryan was one such pillar of encouragement and advice, as has been Terry Cullinane in more recent years. Now working as a secretary in the Department of Oral Health and Development, Terry often organises fund-raisers

BRÍD RYAN:
CLINICAL SECRETARY & FRIEND TO STUDENTS

One of the most beloved figures in the history of the school was its long-time clinical secretary, Bríd Ryan. Born Bríd Cronin, she studied dentistry at UCC, receiving her BDS in 1940. She stood out as a camogie player, winning Ashbourne Cup medals with UCC and a remarkable three all-Ireland camogie medals with Cork (in 1939, 1940 and 1941). In later years, she became a noted golfer. Her athletic background proved helpful when she began her public-health dental career during the 1940s. Bríd's first job required her to travel across Munster providing dental services to patients unable to travel to Cork city at a time when wartime fuel restrictions limited automobile traffic. Carrying a bag of instruments, she cycled from Cork to such towns as Mallow, Bandon, Macroom and Fermoy, treating patients and returning to Cork the same day.

Joining CUDSH in the 1960s as clinical secretary (assuming many of the responsibilities formerly held by the hospital matron), she replaced her bicycle with a Ford Anglia, which she parked in the 'North Cha'. Bríd was very involved in all aspects of the dental hospital, and counted numerous staff members as friends. She possessed a genuine interest in the welfare of the students, whom she took the trouble of knowing individually. Within the hospital, she advocated for patients, ensuring their prompt treatment or explaining their special circumstances to staff. She became a human face for patient and student interactions, a role well-suited to her warm personality.

Bríd remained enormously popular with generations of dental students. She supervised and signed off on the different stages of dental procedures, while frequently enquiring about students' general well-being. At a time of expanding class sizes, she ensured that no one slipped between the cracks. Students have recounted how during an examination when their procedure was not going according to plan, Bríd would covertly signal them to the hand-washing sink. There she would quietly impart some relevant advice to salvage the procedure at hand.

Bríd enjoyed the social side of life at the dental hospital, and acted almost as the unofficial hostess of the annual school dinner dance. With little difficulty, she could be prevailed upon to perform her party piece, 'Scarlet Ribbons'. Her lively sense of humour was often deployed to regale a crowd with stories of past student sagas or staff misadventures.

The Cork University Dental School and Hospital welded her personality strengths with her professional capabilities. Her dental training and manual dexterity made her a valued teaching resource. Her natural people skills and personal generosity enabled her to relate to patients, students and staff to the mutual benefit of all. She mixed charisma with efficiency, making CUDSH a better and more enjoyable place.

Bríd Ryan (right) with Claire Barry, a part-time lecturer in orthodontics at CUDSH from 1971 to 2001.
COURTESY CLAIRE BARRY

for such charities as the Irish Lifeboats and the Arc House, which continues the school's long tradition of supporting worthy causes. One memorable fund-raiser occurred in 1960, when students Pat McDonagh and Pat Kidd pushed a pram from Dublin to Cork. Most of the student body met them as they entered the city. During the centenary year of 2013, dental students led by Joey Donovan organised a golf tournament to support the Cork Dental Outreach Programme. It dispatched eleven students to an impoverished neighbourhood in Nepal, where they provided essential dental care for three weeks. Similar philanthropic efforts have been common throughout the decades at CUDSH.

SPORTS

Though golf remains an occupational hazard for dentists, CUDSH has been associated with other sporting achievements that reflect its social and cultural diversity. Indeed, the first school dean, Hubert O'Keeffe, was a substitute for the Irish rugby team on three occasions, though apparently without once making it onto the field of play. Hubert also hunted and golfed, and was president of the Shandon Boat Club. From such a foundation, the school has produced a string of successful sporting men and women, including seven graduates who performed at international level.

Mary Kiely (BDS 1986) has been a long-time hockey international for Ireland. She was inspired by her grand-aunt Mary Goggin (BDS 1924), who played hockey for Munster. As a goalkeeper, Mary Kiely has served Ireland at all levels. After qualifying, she practised in England and continued to play hockey at county level for Cheshire. She married a dental graduate from her own class (John Bowen), and they currently live in Dungarvan. A clinical dental surgeon with the HSE, she still plays hockey for the Irish senior team.

Serryth Colbert (BDS 2001) rowed for NUI Galway while

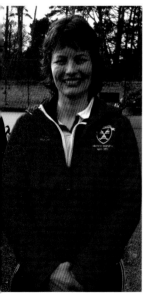

International hockey player, Mary Kiely.
COURTESY MARY KIELY

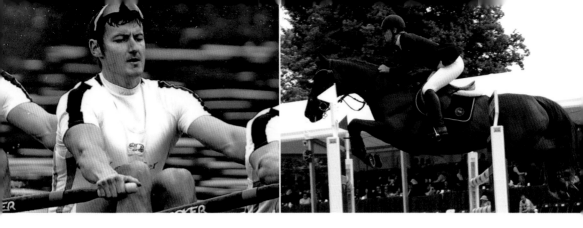

studying medicine, and for UCC while studying dentistry. He won numerous university championships for both colleges, while simultaneously representing Ireland in international competitions. After finishing his BDS, Serryth moved to Britain's famed Leander Club in Henley-on-Thames, where he won three gold medals at the Henley Royal Regatta, numerous British national championships, and a Commonwealth Games gold medal (racing with Team GB). Serryth also rowed with the Irish heavyweight boat in the Athens (2004) and Beijing (2008) Olympic Games. After working full-time in the NHS as a registrar in oral and maxillofacial surgery, he took up a position as the cleft and craniofacial fellow for the south-west of England in July 2013. Serryth authored the fascinating article 'Performing to a world class standard under pressure – can we learn lessons from the Olympians?' for the *British Journal of Oral and Maxillofacial Surgery* (vol. 50 (2012), pp. 291–7). He interviewed forty-three oral surgeons and forty-six Olympic rowers to compare their mental preparations, technical skills and performance under pressure. He found psychology a key factor to achieving success, along with diligent training. The study is regarded as a classic of its type.

At an early age, sisters Sarah-Kate Quinlivan (BDS 2006) and Danielle Quinlivan (BDS 2007) achieved national and international recognition as showjumpers. Sarah-Kate was one of the most successful riders on the national and international junior circuit. As a fourth-year dental student, she broke into the senior circuit, finishing runner-up in the 2005 National Grand Prix and being named Rookie of the Year for the season. She was

(left) International and Olympic rower, Serryth Colbert; (right) international showjumper, Sarah-Kate Quinlivan.

Courtesy Serryth Colbert & Danielle Quinlivan

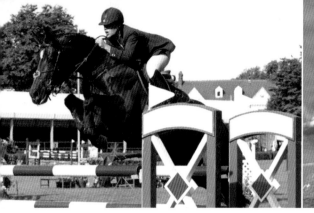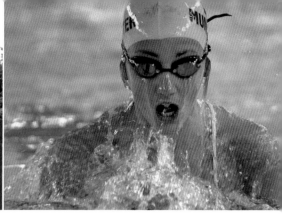

(left) International showjumper Danielle Quinlivan; (right) International modern pentathlete, Sally McCarthy.

COURTESY DANIELLE QUINLIVAN & SALLY MCCARTHY

promptly selected for the senior national showjumping team, whose international competition coincided with her final-year dental studies. School staff (especially Dr Frank Burke) supported her successful application for a one-month leave of absence. The leave subsequently yielded a silver medal in the international team competition in Greece. After completing her BDS the following year, Sarah-Kate was placed in the top ten in the Hickstead Derby in Sussex and in the Dublin Grand Prix. She currently works in general practice in London, and hopes to continue showjumping. Sarah-Kate's sister Danielle likewise progressed through the youth ranks, wining numerous national and international Grand Prix titles, and representing Ireland on cup teams more than twenty times. After her elevation to the senior team, Danielle took a two-year break to undertake cadet training with the Irish Defence Forces. In 1998 she was commissioned as the army's first female riding officer, stationed at the Army Equitation School. In addition to her military duties, Danielle represented Ireland at international competitions in Europe and South America. After leaving the army, she followed her sister to CUDSH. She still competes on the showjumping and eventing circuit during breaks from private practice in Kanturk. Fortunately, she works with her father Michael (BDS 1973), who has been a forgiving practice partner.

One of the school's most impressive athletes is Sally McCarthy (BDS 2011), who enjoyed an extraordinary schoolgirl career. In athletics, she won numerous youth titles in the 1500 and 800 metres. She also played hockey on Munster junior and senior

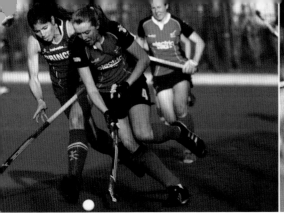
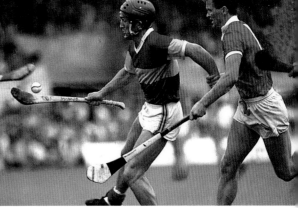

teams, and competed in showjumping. Sally's success reached the water, as she joined the Irish junior women's water polo squad in 2005, and won the 2004 Fastnet International Schools Regatta Topper Fleet. With such talent, she naturally progressed to the modern pentathlon (comprised of running, swimming, shooting, showjumping and fencing) and the Tetrathlon (the same events bar fencing). After taking up fencing, she won the 2009 Irish modern pentathlon ranking title, and represented Ireland while finishing fifth at the Swiss Open. During her fourth year of dentistry, she trained with the 2012 Irish Olympic developmental squad. Unfortunately, she found it too difficult to juggle the two demanding activities, and surrendered her Olympic dream in favour of a BDS degree. After qualifying, Sally moved to England and currently trains with Team Bath on a performance scholarship. She also works part-time in a mixed NHS and private practice.

Miriam Crowley is a final-year dental student for 2013–14. The product of a distinguished Cork sporting family, her father, Tim Crowley, won three All-Ireland senior hurling medals with Cork. Miriam represented Munster in hockey at underage and senior school levels, and played for the Irish U-16s. Entering UCC in 2008, she was called to Ireland's second team, 'Ireland A'. In 2010 Miriam won her first hockey senior international cap against Scotland. She was subsequently selected for the Irish women's hockey-team training programme in Dublin, which met every weekend. The Irish squad selected her to compete in the 2011 European Championships, with top teams advancing to the 2012 Olympic Games in London. She suspended her BDS studies to

(left) International hockey player, Miriam Crowley; (right) Cork All-Ireland hurling winner, Pat Hartnett.

Courtesy Miriam Crowley & Pat Hartnett

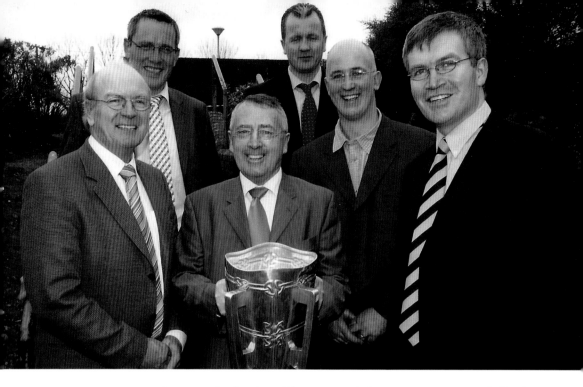

*Cork All-Ireland dentist
hurlers and the Liam
McCarthy Cup during a visit
to the dental hospital, 2002:
(back, left to right) J. Browne,
P. Hartnett;
(front, left to right)
P. Crowley (trainer),
D. O'Mullane, M. Foley,
R. Browne.*

Courtesy Paddy Crowley

focus on the hockey Olympic qualification campaign, a difficult decision made with the blessing of school staff (again supported by Dr Frank Burke). Unfortunately, after a string of victories, the Irish team fell at the last Olympic hurdle, losing a final qualifying match. Denied her Olympic dream, Miriam has resumed her dental studies and will sit her final BDS examination in June 2014. She hopes to continue her international hockey career, which to date has resulted in fifty-six caps.

Cork has produced a number of distinguished dentist hurlers, including Liam Shalloe (BDS 1960), who represented Waterford at senior level for a number of years. Liam, a long-time member of the part-time teaching staff, married his classmate Katherine Moloney (BDS 1960), and their daughter Patricia (BDS 1996) has inherited Liam's periodontology practice in Cork city.

In the annals of Cork hurling, 7 September 1986 was an especially proud day for CUDSH. Cork defeated Kilkenny to win the All-Ireland senior hurling championship. Playing for Cork were two CUDSH graduates, Richard Browne (BDS 1985) and Pat Hartnett (BDS 1995). Richard enjoyed a fruitful hurling career with UCC, winning the 1985 Fitzgibbon Cup on a panel that included a number of fellow dental students. The year 1986 was memorable for Richard, as he qualified for his BDS and won Munster and All-Ireland senior hurling medals with Cork. He served the county at senior level from 1986 to 1991. Pat Hartnett played with Cork between 1984 and 1994, winning All-Ireland senior medals in 1984 and 1986. After qualifying, Pat secured an M.Sc. (Cons) from Eastman, University of London, and now works in private specialist practice in Cork city. Timoleague native Mark Foley (BDS 1989) joined the Cork senior team in 1990, and is still remembered for that year's Munster championship against Tipperary, when he was named man of the match after scoring a remarkable two goals and seven points from play. He won one All-Ireland title, and played in a second All-Ireland final that ended in defeat. He is currently in practice in Bantry, County Cork. John Browne (BDS 2000) emerged from Blackrock and UCC to secure a place on the

CUDSH staff soccer team early 1960s: (back, left to right) S. O'Donovan, unknown, L. O'Connell, B. Barrett, T. O'Riordan, R. O'Neill; (front, left to right) N. Cronin, D. O'Mullane, J. Kenefick, L. Shalloe.
COURTESY JOE HALLISSEY

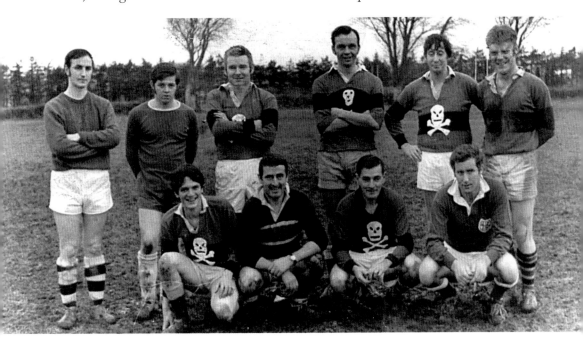

inter-county team from 1998 to 2004. In 1999 he helped Cork beat Kilkenny in the All-Ireland final, and came on as a substitute in the 2004 final, which he played without a helmet. An outstanding hurler, John was renowned for his coolness under pressure.

In camogie, Claire Cronin (née Murphy) has been outstanding at inter-county level, as well as a valued member of the clinical-teaching staff at the Dental Hygiene School. Having begun her career at St Aloysius Secondary School in Cork, Claire won a remarkable four senior All-Ireland medals (in 1978, 1980, 1982 and 1983) playing with the Cork senior camogie team. In doing so, she followed in the footsteps of the popular dental-hospital staff member Bríd Ryan (née Cronin, BDS 1940). While studying dentistry at UCC, Bríd emerged as a skilled hockey and camogie player. She won three All-Ireland camogie medals with Cork in 1939, 1940 and 1941.

Charlie Teehan (BDS 1950) was born in Buttevant, County Cork, in 1919, and played in three rugby internationals for Ireland in 1939 (against England, Scotland and Wales). A prop forward, his international career ended prematurely with the outbreak of the Second World War. While serving with British forces, he was evacuated from Dunkirk and later joined the Royal Air Force as a rear gunner. Back in Cork, he enjoyed a colourful student career in which he was remembered as a man among boys. Charlie later practised dentistry in the north of England. Boyle Cussen (BDS 1958) was a talented wing forward with UCC and Munster, playing on the famous 1954 Munster team that narrowly lost to the New Zealand All Blacks at the Mardyke. Also on the pitch was Robin Godfrey, who later served as secretary of the UCC Medical Faculty. UCC dentist Charlie Haly (BDS 1995) starred in Munster's celebrated victory against Australia in 1992. At full back in Musgrave Park that day (he also played on the wings), Charlie kicked fourteen points to pull Munster clear by a final score of 22 to 19. He also played for Oxford while a postgraduate studying economics and politics. His father, Mick Haly, was a highly regarded part-time lecturer in the Department of Anatomy during the 1960s and 1970s. Charlie is currently in private practice in Cork city.

Such activities by CUDSH students and graduates reflect a larger sporting tradition at UCC, recently exemplified by the university's appointment of Declan Kidney (former coach of the Irish national rugby team) as director of sport and physical activity. It can also be noted that at the All-Ireland hurling final played on 8 September 2013, twenty-seven out of fifty players, trainers and coaches from Cork and Clare had UCC links.

One former Cork student deserves special recognition for non-sports achievement. Majella Cullagh completed her dental-nursing training at CUDSH, and as a student regularly performed at musical events throughout the city. Spotted by Maeve Coughlan at the Cork School of Music, she won a scholarship to the National Opera Studio in London and studied with the famous Gerald Martin Moore. Since the 1990s, Majella has regularly performed a wide repertoire ranging from Handel and Mozart to Donizetti, Rossini and Verdi. She has worked with such acclaimed conductors as Macarus, Tate and Corella, and directors such as Zambello, Savera and Halls. Her magnificent voice can be heard on the Opera Rara label, and in great opera houses around the world.

DENTAL GRADUATES HOME & AWAY

Many CUDSH graduates have made major contributions to dentistry nationally and internationally. Some notable examples can be offered.

Bill Murphy (BDS 1957) was born in Clonmel, County Tipperary, and served as a dental officer in various general and dental hospitals following graduation. After completing his fellowship in the Royal College of Surgeons in England in 1960,

STUDENTS, SHOWBANDS & 'THE DINOSAURS'

During the mid-1960s Cork dental students calling themselves 'The Dinosaurs' brought popular musical acts into Cork city. They played a supporting role during Ireland's celebrated showband era, at a time when young people experienced growing social liberation.

In the 1960s student life revolved around dances, which were inexpensive opportunities to interact with the opposite sex. Musical appreciation grew with the arrival of pirate radio (unlicensed radio stations usually devoted to rock and roll). This created a high demand for live music venues that allowed dancing.

Weekend dance cards filled up quickly. The Refinery Club (on Alfred Street) attracted students on Friday nights, as did the Gresham Rooms on Maylor Street. Saturdays (the main night out) featured dances at the Cork Constitution clubhouse, the Cork Boat Club, the Lee Boat Club, and the Shandon Boat Club. Sundays catered specifically to UCC students, with a regular dance held on campus at the Main Rest (the student restaurant). However, a clear void existed midweek. A group of dental students – John Barry (BDS 1966), Robin Power (BDS 1967) and Eddie Kenneally (BDS 1967) – and a medical student, Jack Cantillon, decided to fill that gap with a designated student dance. They called themselves The Dinosaurs.

After struggling for a year to find a regular venue (Cork City Hall proved difficult to reserve), they fixed a weekly dance at the Arcadia hall. Located on the Lower Road, 'The Arc' was owned by the Prendergast family and could accommodate eighteen hundred people. The Dinosaurs booked the talent, promoted the dances, and sold tickets, while Arcadia staff worked the door, bar and cloakroom. In 1965 Wednesday became student night at The Arc, with a non-alcoholic dance running from 9 pm to 1 am. Strict bouncers virtually eradicated disturbances inside. The Prendergasts accurately predicted that middle-class university students would help draw a large but 'respectable' crowd. The Dinosaurs profited from ticket sales, while the Arcadia soaked up money at the non-alcoholic mineral bar.

Students heard Ireland's most popular showbands, usually covering pop and rock hits. These included famous acts like The Royal Showband, Joe Dolan, The Freshmen, The Miami Showband and Cork's most beloved export, The Dixies. According to John Barry, performers were chosen on the basis of 'who would draw a crowd'. The Dinosaurs printed posters and placed newspaper advertisements, and otherwise creatively filled the hall. With the Arcadia located at the opposite end of Cork from the university, The Dinosaurs hired buses to carry students to and from Bishopstown, Douglas and UCC. Students and hospital nurses received reduced ticket rates, an innovation at the time. The dance was open to all third-level students, not just those from UCC, thereby drawing students from the local technical college and the schools of commerce and music. When students went home for the summer, The Dinosaurs drew crowds by holding raffles and prune-eating and fancy-dress competitions. Their most popular dance of the year was Shrove Tuesday, which they billed as 'the last chance to meet a girl before Lent'.

The Dinosaur ran dances for eight years, but ultimately fell victim to competing career demands and boredom. During that time, the student entrepreneurs earned enough to pay their dental-school fees, and to buy their own automobiles, an unheard of luxury at the time. They left behind memories of thumping stages, sweltering dance floors and cool cycles home with someone draped across the handlebars. It was a time of some innocence, though not as much as contemporary readers are often led to believe.

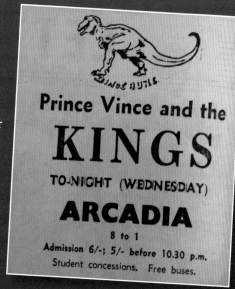

he obtained his MDS degree from Newcastle Upon Tyne. There he became a lecturer in prosthetic dentistry, before taking up a lecturing and professorial position in the School of Dentistry at Cardiff University. He served on numerous national and international dental bodies, and published more than fifty refereed articles, mainly in dental prosthetics.

Terry English (BDS 1959) first qualified in medicine before passing his BDS. He then took up a house-officer position in Eastman Dental Hospital in London, specialising in oral and maxillofacial surgery. The first dentist awarded a diploma at the Royal College of Surgeons in Dublin, Terry was recruited by Professor Sir Terrence Ward to the world-famous plastic-surgery unit in Queen Victoria Hospital, Sussex. Established by Sir Archibald McIndoe in 1941, it specifically treated war pilots who had sustained severe burns to their face and hands. McIndoe and Ward's plastic-surgery techniques restored the facial appearance of many severely disfigured pilots, allowing them to return to a relatively normal life. Patients recuperated in East Grinstead, which became known as 'the town that doesn't stare'. After that experience, Terry moved to the Oral and Maxillofacial Unit at the Royal London Hospital, Whitechapel. He married Una Atkins, a UCC medical graduate and the daughter of UCC president Henry St John Atkins.

Brian O'Riordan (BDS 1958) is the son of Paddy O'Riordan (BDS 1925). Brian was auditor of the UCC Dental Student Society in 1957 when it produced the dental-school tie and scarf from a design by Michael Dunne (BDS 1961). After qualification, Brian held oral-surgery posts at various hospitals in the London area before obtaining the Fellowship of the Royal College of Surgeons of England. He became an oral-surgery consultant at the Central Middlesex Hospital and at the Plastic and Jaw Surgery Centre in Northwood, Middlesex, in 1970. Two years later, he was appointed a consultant in dental radiology at King's College School of Medicine and Dentistry. As a postgraduate tutor, he ran the first course for the MGDS RCS (Eng.) diploma. He has been a leader within various professional associations: he was treasurer of the British Association of Oral Surgeons, and in 1981 became president of the British Association of Oral and Maxillofacial Radiology. Beyond dentistry, Brian is a liveryman of the Worshipful Company of Glaziers and Painters of Glass, and in 2013 became a Freeman of the City of London.

Eugene David Vaughan (BDS 1967) served from 1995 to 2009 as senior surgeon at Aintree University Hospital, Liverpool. Internationally recognised in his field, Dr Vaughan was president of the British Association of Oral and Maxillofacial Surgeons in 2002, and president of the British Association of Head & Neck Oncologists from 2005 to 2007.

Dr Anne Aiken (née Whelton) (BDS 1970) found success in London. After qualifying, she was a house surgeon for a year in the old dental hospital, before undertaking orthodontic training at Eastman Dental Hospital and the Royal Dental Hospital. She served as a registrar under Brian O'Riordan at Middlesex Hospital, before moving to The London Hospital (now Barts and The London), where she eventually became a senior lecturer and honorary consultant. She continued her research while becoming a key member of the school's teaching staff. Along the way, she completed a Ph.D. in oral and maxillofacial surgery. Active in the Royal College of Surgeons, England, she received an honorary Fellowship of Dental Surgery (FDS) in recognition of her contributions to that body (she had already secured an FDS from RCS Edinburgh in 1975). Upon her retirement in 2002, Dr Aiken moved to the British judiciary. Currently, she sits as a non-stipendiary magistrate in North West London.

Robin O'Sullivan (BDS 1971) qualified in both dentistry and medicine at UCC. He lectured in the UCC Anatomy Department from 1978 to 2004. His M.Sc. and Ph.D. research dealt with ultrastructural aspects of the peripheral nervous system, and he gained extensive teaching experience in anatomy, histology, embryology and anthropology. Moving to the Middle East in 2004, he taught at Jordan University of Science and Technology and at Kuwait University. Currently, he is professor of anatomy and chairman of the Department of Basic Medical Sciences at RCSI Bahrain. His current research focus is enamel structure and historical biography, though he maintains an interest in anatomy. (See the O'Sullivan Dynasty, below.)

Nuala Porteous (née Walsh) (BDS 1975) worked seven years in private practice before obtaining a Master of Public Health from the University of Texas Health Science Center at Houston. She has since become an associate professor at the San Antonio Dental School, attached to the same centre. Dr Porteous specialises in infection-control issues, and has published extensively on dental-unit waterline contamination.

Peter Cooney (BDS 1977) moved to Canada, where he completed advanced degrees in community dentistry. After service with First Nation and Inuit communities in Manitoba, he was appointed Canada's first chief dental officer. Dr Cooney has remained in that position since 2004, and stays active in international dental public-health bodies. He is a past president of the Canadian Association of Public Health Dentistry, and a former chief examiner with the Royal College of Dentists of Canada.

Dr Patrick J. Byrne (BDS 1982) held various hospital appointments from 1982 to 1989. In 1990 he completed his M.Sc. in periodontology at the Eastman Dental Institute, and was awarded the Sir Wilfred Fish Research Prize by the British Society of Periodontology. He has served in multiple lecturing posts since then, and gained numerous distinguished qualifications. Joining the Faculty of Dentistry, Royal College of Surgeons in Ireland, he was its dean from 2007 until 2011.

After qualifying from Cork with first-class honours, Brian O'Connell (BDS 1984) trained in prosthodontics and biochemistry at the Eastman Dental Center, University of Rochester, New York. There he made an immediate impact as a clinician and an award-winning researcher. He continued his research at the National Institute of Dental and Craniofacial Research in Bethesda, Maryland. Currently, Brian is professor of restorative dentistry at Trinity College Dublin, where he works on prosthodontics, and oral health and aging.

Gerard Bradley (BDS 1988) completed a three-year residence in orthodontics at Ohio State University. A specialist in ortho-dontic materials and clinical outcomes, he is currently professor, programme director and department chairman at the Marquette University School of Dentistry.

Seán McCarthy (BDS 1989) also pursued an advanced degree in the United States. He completed a three-year postgraduate programme in prosthodontics at the Louisiana State University School of Dentistry. He spent another year there as a teaching fellow, and subsequently became a diplomat for the American Board of Prosthodontics. Seán returned to Cork in 2000 to open a referral-based practice, and co-authored (with Finbarr Allen) *Complete Dentures: From Planning to Problem Solving* (Quintessentials Series).

Five distinguished CUDSH postgraduates can be mentioned, each of whom was supervised by Denis O'Mullane. Dublin product Dr John Clarkson completed his Ph.D. at Cork in 1987, before becoming executive director of the International Association for Dental Research, headquartered in the United States. He was sub-sequently elected president of that body, one of two Cork graduates to hold that notable position (Helen Whelton is the other). Dr Clarkson returned to Ireland to take up the chair of dental public health in the Dublin Dental University and Hospital, and is now emeritus professor there. Professor Ailish Hannigan completed a Ph.D. in biostatistics at CUDSH. She is currently professor of biomedical statistics at the University of Limerick Medical School.

Professor Roger Ellwood was the clinical examiner of the North Wales Schoolchildren Study undertaken by the Oral Health Services Research Centre, and received his Ph.D. from UCC in 1988. Currently, he is head of research in the Oral Healthcare Division of Colgate-Palmolive, and honorary professor of dental diagnostic science at the University of Manchester School of Dentistry. Professor Jacinta MacLoughlin of the School of Dental Science at TCD earned her Master of Dental Science degree at CUDSH. A member of the Dental Council of Ireland, she has published extensively. Her husband Ambrose is secretary general of the Department of Health and Children. An oral-health researcher and dentist who qualified in Dublin, he received his MBA at UCC. Both Ambrose and Jacinta obtained their BDent SC degrees at TCD.

Finally, a history of the Cork University Dental School and Hospital would be incomplete without mentioning Ray Gamble (BDS 1933). He enjoyed a long career as a general practitioner, obtained an FFDRCSI, and taught at the school from 1936 to 1976. Ray also served on the Fluoride Consultative Council established by the minister for health in 1957. That body's recommendations resulted in the passage of the Health (Fluoridation of Water Supplies) Act, 1960. In 1982 Ray published *History of the Cork Dental Hospital and School from 1913–1982*, which has proved an essential text and reference during the writing of this book. He was a dedicated servant to the school and hospital.

DENTAL DYNASTIES

When considering a hundred years of dental graduates, the frequency of familial connections becomes clear. It is difficult to determine the exact cause of this continuity, though social, economic and cultural reasons are all likely factors. Among the school alumni, some notable siblings and multigenerational pairings are visible.

THE EGANS/O'MEARAS

Louis J. Egan was a registered dentist who co-founded CUDSH in 1913. His son, also Louis Egan, practised as a dentist in the city, while his daughter was the mother of two more UCC dental graduates. Her son James (Jim) O'Meara (BDS 1924) set up practice in Mallow and became the first Cork graduate to be elected president of the Irish Dental Association. Charles (Charlie) O'Meara (BDS 1926) practised in Fermoy. Two of Charlie O'Meara's sons also qualified in dentistry: David (BDS 1959) and Michael (BDS 1966). David took over his father's Fermoy practice, and Michael established a new one in Mitchelstown. David's son Cian (BDS 2006) joined his father's practice in Fermoy, and Michael's son Marcus (BDS Dundee 1999) is currently in dental practice in Australia.

THE OLLIVERES

Joseph Francis Ollivere apprenticed to a dentist working at Charing Cross Road in 1865, and joined the first Dental Register in 1878. At that time, he was believed to be practising at 10 Cook Street, Cork. His son, Thomas Joseph Ollivere LDS, co-founded CUDSH in 1913. He practised at 60 South Mall, and his name is still visible on its letter box. Thomas Joseph's son Joseph Denis Francis Ollivere (BDS 1938) became the first Cork graduate to receive a Higher Diploma in Dentistry (HDD) from the Royal College of Surgeons, Edinburgh. He worked in practice at 60 South Mall, and served on the dental-hospital staff from 1940 to 1953. Joseph accepted a dental lectureship at the University of Malaya in Singapore, before returning in 1961 to become a lecturer at the School of Dental Hygiene in the Royal Dental Hospital, London. His son Peter Thomas Robert Ollivere qualified at the Royal Dental Hospital, London, in 1972. After twenty-five years in the Royal Air Force Dental Corps, he is currently in orthodontic practice in Eastbourne.

THE O'SULLIVANS

The O'Sullivan dynasty has been linked with Cork dentistry for five generations. The connection began with Tommy Hill, who in 1885 completed his dental apprenticeship with 'Kippy' Goldfoot, reportedly the first Jewish dentist in Cork. Tommy's daughter Evelyn Maud Hill married Denis O'Sullivan, Tommy's own apprentice. Denis O'Sullivan and Evelyn Maud had a son, Cecil O'Sullivan (BDS 1945), who ran a successful general practice in Dunbar Street, Cork, for over forty years. His son Robin O'Sullivan (BDS Cork 1971) qualified in both dentistry and medicine at UCC. Like her father, Robin's daughter Emma (BDS 2000) studied dentistry and medicine. She is currently completing specialist training in oral and maxillofacial surgery in Scotland.

More than one former staff member has described the Cork University Dental School and Hospital as 'like a family'. As can be seen from Cork's notable dental families, in many cases this can be taken literally. Ultimately, such familial networks add another layer to the institution's vibrant dental community. They illustrate the dynamic nature of CUDSH connections, which frequently return to regenerate the institution.

Having begun in Cork city's South Mall, the Cork University Dental School and Hospital extended its reach first to the rest of Munster and then to Ireland. Subsequently, its dentists could be found across Britain and, later, throughout the English-speaking world. Today, that dental community has become global. Its dentists, teachers, nurses, dental hygienists and researchers practise their craft on six continents, maintaining the professional standards they learned in Cork.

EPILOGUE:
THE NEXT HUNDRED YEARS

ONE hundred years after its founding, the Cork University Dental School and Hospital has become a vibrant oral-health-care, research and educational centre. It annually produces between forty and forty-five BDS graduates, along with fourteen dental hygienists, and thirty-five to forty dental nurses (graduating every eighteen months). There are currently nineteen registered Ph.D. students, evenly split between the school and the Oral Health Research Centre. Each department continues to train students pursuing higher specialist training programmes, master's degrees and diplomas. CUDSH employs ninety-nine full-time members of staff.

School administrators envision certain growth areas in the near future. Students will receive more-intense instruction on professional, legal and ethical issues (a need first recognised in the 1950s, when students took courses in sociology, psychology and philosophy). Similarly, practical aspects of dental treatment will be emphasised, such as improving communication skills with patients. The teaching of treatment options will depend on a more valid evidence base. The school anticipates the continued evolution of electronic technology, which will enable students to become lifelong learners. Computer-based simulations will likely change instruction methods, as will the use of portable electronic devices in continuous assessment, and the creation of electronic logbooks. Patient records may become exclusively electronic and incorporate digital-imaging technology. Yet fundamental aspects of dental education will remain unchanged. Teaching staff will continue to verify students' clinical competence by assessing their treatment of patients. Graduates will still be clinically accomplished. Many will develop the skills necessary to progress to senior leadership positions in dentistry.

As people are living longer and keeping their natural teeth for much longer in life, a much broader dental workforce will be needed. Dental education must recognise that dentists cannot be proficient in all aspects of oral health care. Care delivery requires a team approach, as opposed to the traditional single-handed-practitioner model.

The education of all members of the dental team will likely undergo substantial change in the next ten to twenty years. Undergraduate dental-curriculum emphasis will shift away from creating competence in all primary dental-care procedures, and towards developing more-advanced expertise in clinical leadership, risk assessment, advanced information technology, diagnosis and treatment planning. This will allow other members of the dental team to make fuller contributions to oral-health-care provision. All members of the dental team will be involved in a lifelong continuum of education, possibly involving periods of retraining. An increasing number of dental graduates will continue on to the masters level to develop advanced knowledge and skills in areas in which they have particular interests or abilities. Such individuals will probably seek to work in multi-surgery practices or dental centres in which shared patient care is the norm.

By the end of the current decade, there will be a new legislative framework for dentistry, and it will be described as a Dental Act as opposed to the existing Dentists' Act. The new Dental Act will regulate not just dentists but also other dental-care professionals (DCPs), such as dental hygienists, dental therapists and clinical-dental technicians. The team approach to dental care will influence DCP courses offered at CUDSH, with new degree programmes likely to replace the current diplomas. DCP programmes will better align with BDS programmes, and they will be subjected to a similarly high scholarly rigour, to be monitored by the Dental Council of Ireland. Dental-hospital services will be reconfigured to provide sufficient patients for the training of all DCP students, which will impact on hospital infrastructure and staffing. It is hoped that the Department of Health and Children will provide the necessary funding to train Irish students in these areas.

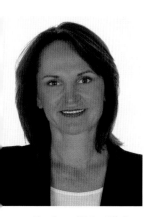

Professor Helen Whelton, director of OHSRC (2006–13), recently appointed dean, Leeds Dental Institute, University of Leeds.
Courtesy CUDSH

In the coming years, it is likely that the number of recognised specialities and the pattern of their training regimes will expand. Current Irish postgraduate dental training is almost exclusively privately funded, which limits access. A further challenge to post-graduates is the lack of a clear career structure. Dental graduates will likely continue to seek postgraduate training opportunities abroad, and then attempt to return to private specialist practice in Ireland. Owing to the high cost of specialist training and the need for a cadre of qualified instructors, the situation can only be modified by a new public policy and service-delivery model. A fresh policy direction will undoubtedly increase the number of taught postgraduate trainees.

Currently, there are exciting research opportunities on the horizon. A major growth area will be found in the development of information technology to facilitate surgical planning and the manufacture of dental prostheses. Stem-cell research is also an important area, while the ability to differentiate dental tissues and grow teeth will necessitate major investigation. Though in some ways this work is in its early days, its potential is exciting.

UCC has emphasised the need for world-class research at the university. Though CUDSH has made major research contributions (see Chapter 5), continued progress will require significantly more time and financial investment. Research has reached a cross-roads at CUDSH. The present fiscal climate has made it more difficult to balance research with teaching and clinical treatment. The lack of a promotional scheme for researchers is a major barrier, as is a shortage of qualified candidates (part of a global trend). Research enhances clinical teaching and benefits the broader community, which makes its proper funding and staffing a pressing institutional priority. It is hoped that these challenges will merit a serious discussion by professional, academic and state stakeholders.

The next century will likely produce as many challenges as the previous one. With this in mind, certain institutional changes may be necessary. In 2011 Professor John Higgins, head of the College of Medicine and Health, invited Alf Smiddy and Professor Cillian Twomey to conduct an independent review of the Cork University Dental School and Hospital so as to assess its governance in relation to patient service, teaching and research. Their findings provide a number of points for reflection and signposts for future roads ahead. The report recognises the limitations of its current governance, which resulted from organic growth during the past three decades. Unlike other Irish hospitals and health-care research centres, CUDSH is managed by its faculty, who answer directly to University College Cork. Such a structure was intended to be temporary, though it has remained in place since 1968. School authorities envision the institution as an academic health centre for dentistry. As such, it should be managed by representatives of UCC, relevant health services and the community at large. Additional and more imaginative leadership structures will ensure the creation and implementation of a sustainable strategy for the future.

Financially, CUDSH has retained its long-standing cost-efficiency. However, the existing funding model does not generate enough revenue to accommodate a budget in line with similarly sized dental institutions in Europe. Nationally, CUDSH maintains roughly the same educational outputs as the Dublin dental hospital (similar undergraduate levels, but Dublin produces more postgraduates). However, Cork's budget is less than half that of Dublin's (the figures for the year ending September 2011 were €9,618,138 for Cork against €23,720,520 for Dublin). While the Dublin dental hospital has enjoyed certain structural advantages, it has also produced significant revenue by delivering dental services to a number of public constituencies. In Cork, the expansion of service-level agreements between the HSE and CUDSH would improve the latter's financial situation and reinforce its long-standing commitment to serving its community.

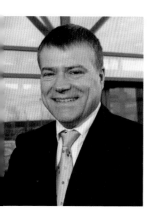

Professor Finbarr Allen, dean CUDSH, 2007–13.
Courtesy CUDSH

The 'new' dental hospital is already thirty-one years old, based on a forty-year-old design. Though the hospital functions well at the moment, there is little space for new instruments or treatment facilities likely to appear in the near future. One can easily envision a circumstance similar to the last days of the old hospital, with modern equipment jammed into spaces not purpose-built for it. It will be essential for the dental hospital to secure enough room to expand as emerging needs are identified.

Cork University Hospital has recently sought new land to accommodate a major expansion. The property occupied by the Cork University Dental School and Hospital and the Oral Health Service Research Centre would enable such growth. Preliminary discussions have been held about relocating the entire dental school and hospital and the OHSRC to the South Infirmary–Victoria University Hospital, located in the city centre near Cork City Hall. The co-location of CUDSH with the South Infirmary would satisfy a core requirement. The new property would also apparently offer additional space for future growth. As such, it is a viable alternative, though the move would require significant public investment. Recalling the saga involving the construction of the current dental hospital at Wilton, school officials will approach any proposals carefully.

Such an undertaking would likely reignite the national debate over the retention of one or two dental schools in Ireland. Students of Irish dental history will recognise a clear advantage to maintaining two dental schools. The Dublin and Cork dental schools have enjoyed healthy competition over the years, and have often generated different models of dental teaching, treatment and research. Each school has learned from the other. The elimination of that institutional competition would likely damage internal innovation and entrepreneurship apparent in the histories of both schools. Observers have attributed much of the current financial crisis to the 'group think' in Ireland's banking and public-finance sectors that produced disastrous policies; a similar danger in dental education and research would be avoided by retaining two separate schools. Locating two dental hospitals in different regions of the country also provides the public-health sector with flexible and robust treatment options. Oral health is an essential part of health care in this country, and should be resourced as such. The public should see the two dental hospitals as a necessity rather than a luxury.

However, the state's two separate dental-education institutions need not operate without reference to one another. From 1938 to 1963, both TCD and UCC shared the teaching services of the imminent orthodontists Dr E. Sheldon Friel and Professor Rodney Dockrell. The National Dental Nurse Training Programme of Ireland, established in 2004 by the Cork and Dublin dental schools, offers another example of cooperation. Two schools should be able to maintain their independence while sharing select services of special consultants or access to expensive new equipment. Closer cooperation between the two institutions could yield better results for both their students and their patients.

Bertram Windle and twelve Cork dentists gathered in a South Mall office a century ago to launch a new dental school. Its mission statement was later listed as 'advancing oral health through excellence and innovation in education, patient care and research'. As dedicated dental educators pursued this goal, they have often faced challenges that seemed insurmountable. In certain periods, the school's future appeared bleak. Yet Cork's dental faculty persevered. Ultimately, they built a modern school and hospital, which was described in 2012 by the consultants Alf Smiddy and Cillian Twomey as follows:

> It has an excellent reputation as an education and training institution; its dental qualifications are highly regarded and its graduates compare very favourably from other dental schools in these islands and beyond.

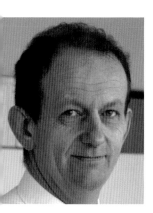

Professor Martin Kinirons, current dean.
Courtesy CUDSH

That Cork University Dental School and Hospital has made significant contributions to national and international dentistry is widely recognised. Its high reputation rests on contributions from generations of diligent teachers, staff, researchers, graduates and friends of the institution. They have constructed a dental-school community that is large, diverse, interconnected and intellectually wealthy. While that community remains healthy, CUDSH will thrive. However, one cannot survive without the other.

The school community has left a rich legacy to a new generation of dental professionals. It is within their power to maintain and ultimately to surpass the institution's achievements in dental education, research and patient treatment. This book's authors sincerely hope they will find the inspiration and the opportunity to do so during the next hundred years.

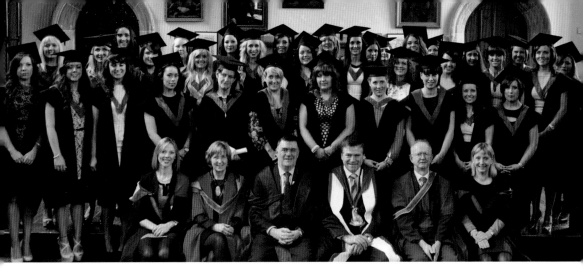

Centenary class, dental-nursing diploma: (back, left to right) Laura O' Donnell, Joanne Foley, Lynsey Parker, Marie Fuller, Sharon Prenderville, Amy Stuart, Ciara Hendy, Chloe Sheehan, Olivia Hickey, Susan Toner, Fiona Kelly, Jacinta Healy, Melissa Waring, Linda Wharton, Marie Kelly, Isobel Fenton, Aoife O'Sullivan, Jennifer Kiely, Ciara O'Brien, Kate McCarthy, Yvonne O'Connell, Celine O'Flynn, Denise Madden;
(centre, left to right) Emma Murphy, Alayne Berkery, Aoife Breen, Alma Clohessy, Louise Coughlan, Michelle Connolly, Emer Coughlan, Margaret Cosgrave, Ruth Delaney, Charlotte Downing, Claire Palmer;
(front, left to right) Siobhán Shakeshaft, Dr Eleanor O'Sullivan, Dr Frank Burke, Professor Finbarr Allen, Dr Noel Ray, Mary Harrington. COURTESY: BARRY'S PHOTOGRAPHIC SERVICES

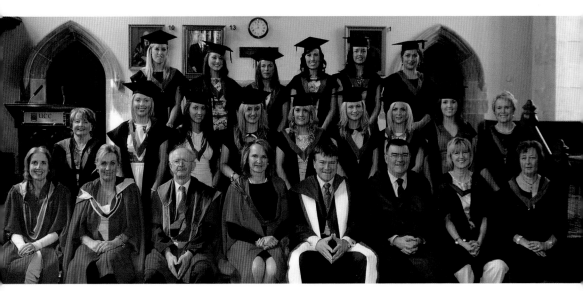

Centenary class, dental-hygiene diploma: (back, left to right) C. Mullins, G. Shannon, M. Madden, A.M. Flannery, A.R. Drumm, M. Cotter; (centre, left to right) Ms A. Holohan, J. O'Riordan, S. Walsh, C. O'Callaghan, N. Kelly, S. Heaney, C. French, R. Cafferkey, Ms C. Murphy;
(front, left to right) Dr O. Barry, Dr S. Curtin, Dr N. Ray, Prof. H. Whelton, Prof. F. Allen, Dr F. Burke, Ms A. O'Keeffe, Ms M. Collins. COURTESY: BARRY'S PHOTOGRAPHIC SERVICES

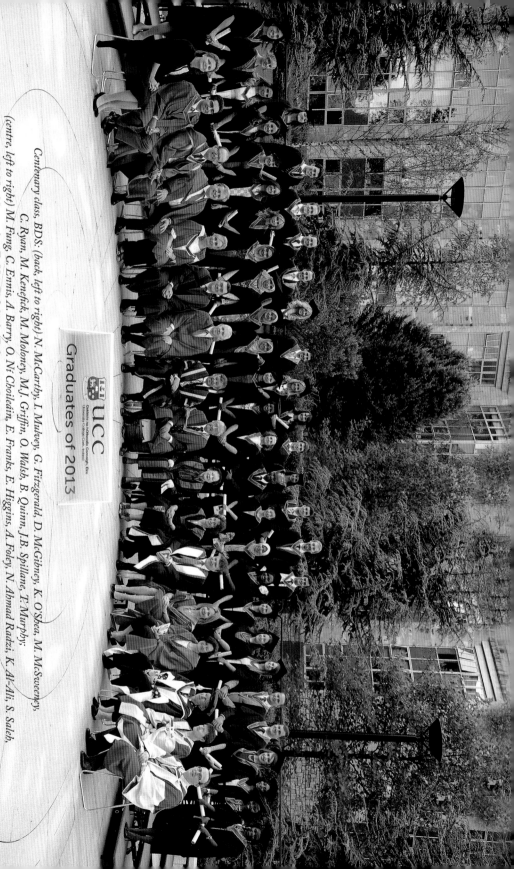

Graduates of 2013

Centenary class, BDS: (back, left to right) N. McCarthy, I. Mulvey, G. Fitzgerald, D. McGibney, K. O'Shea, M. McSweeney,
C. Ryan, M. Kenefick, M. Moloney, M.J. Griffin, O. Walsh, B. Quinn, J.B. Spillane, T. Murphy;
(centre, left to right) M. Fung, C. Ennis, A. Barry, O. Ní Choileáin, E. Franks, E. Higgins, A. Foley, N. Ahmad Radzi, K. Al-Ali, S. Saleh,
H. Nor Nasarudin, E. Hii, B. Odirile, F. Connors, M. Kgosi, M. Cbia, T. Tan Razak, K. Magrudu, N. Coffey, L. Walsh,
A. O'Herlihy, S. Sweetnam, G. Nugent, A. Stack, T. Chacko, R. Mokgosi, D. Ratshipa;
(front, left to right) Dr M. Harding, Dr A. Theocharopoulos, Prof. M. Kinirons, Dr K. Doran, Dr S. Curtin, Dr F. Burke, Prof. J. Higgins, Dr M. Murphy, Prof. D. O'Mullane,
Prof. M. Hegarty, Ms L. Horgan, Prof. F. Allen, Dr E. Allen, Dr C. McCreary, Prof. C. O'Driscoll, Dr S. Byrne. Courtesy: Barry's Photographic Services

APPENDICES

BDS GRADUATES

1915
William Foley
Eugene Whelan

1916
Patrick O'Regan

1917
Edward Murphy

1918
James Lynch
Timothy Nunan
Mary O'Connor
Louis O'Mahony
Daniel O'Mahony
John Wren

1919
Benjamin Birkhahn
Benjamin Brosnan
Ernest O'Shea
Michael Roche

1920
D.P. O'Sullivan
H.M. Horgan

1921
Hannah Horgan
Frank Williams

1923
David O'Driscoll
Richard Twomey
Roland Gallagher

1924
James Breen
Ellen Goggin
Timothy Murphy
James O'Meara
John O'Mahony
Francis Shanahan

1925
John Hayes
Denise Quinlan
William Wren
Mary Clarke
Francis Ferguson
Nicholas Kearney
Patrick Riordan
John Desmond
John A. O'Sullivan

1926
Charles O'Meara
Arthur O'Shea
Angela Pomeroy
Henry Quinlan
Daniel White

1928
Timothy Colbert
Hannah Murphy
Henry Newman
Denis Sweeney

1929
Mary Whelton

1933
Raymond Gamble
Michael Foley

1935
Percy Gremson
Norman Newman

1936
C Wilke

1937
Margaret Keating

1938
Barry Collins
Joseph Ollivere

1940
Brid Cronin
William Cusack
Ita MacCarthy

1941
Mary Barry
Eric Scher

1942
John Long

1943
Harold Newman
Gerald Scher

1944
Leslie Scher
Timothy Clifford
Abraham Khan
Eugene MacSweeney

1945
Cecil O'Sullivan

1946
Aylmer Barrett
Patrick Gleeson
William Gavin

1947
Edward Cashin
James Ryan

1948
Muriel Barry
Desmond Gleeson
John Markham
Patrick O'Donoghue
Mary Gilleran
Mary Keating
James Murray
William Palmer

1949
Elizabeth O'Connell

1950
Patrick Ahern
Eta Crowley
Irene Gallagher
John Hefferman
Margaret Henehan
Daniel Lynch
William Nolan
Patrick O'Sullivan

1951
David Birkhahn
Liam O'Flynn
Mary O'Leary
Henry Murphy
Jeremiah Power
John G. Russell
Ivor Scher
Charles Shinkwin

1952
Robert Ludwig Murphy
Kathleen O'Brien
Philomena Shalvey
Joseph Tynan
John Whelan
Jeremiah Power
Jerome Noel
Mary Roche
William Murphy
Mary Crofts
Turlough O'Brien
Mary Philpott
Jerome Ronayne

1953
Norman Butler
Michael Costello
Christopher Collins
Michael Foley
James McHale
Neil McCann

1954
Patrick Joyce
Denis O'Sullivan
Justin Kidney
Sheila Henry
Desmond Sutherland
John MacSweeney
Elizabeth Shinkwin

1955
Sheila Aherne
Benjamin Attwood
Colm Bell
Thomas Cahill
Mary Connors
Thomas Duggan
Patrick Elwood
Gerald FitzGerald
Jeremiah Healy

Francis Gilligan
Daniel MacDonnell
Francis McGrath
John Murphy
Michael Murray
Nuala Saunders
Patrick Smith
Seamus O'Donoghue
Charles Tehan

1956
Angela Eveline Anthony
Daniel Joyce
John O'Sullivan
Richard Mahony
Redmond F. Walsh
Thomas Wrixon

1957
Vincent Bluett
Louis Buckley
Denis Coffey
Dominic Crofts
Michael Fitzpatrick
Charles Haly
Mary Healy
Una Heskin
Thomas Kelly
Joseph Le Masney
Brendan Long
William Murphy
Patrick Horgan
John Shea
Nora Twomey

continued over

1958
Niall Coakley
Edward Cussen
Josephine Raphael Devlin
Terrence English
Liam Liddy
Liam O'Connell
Jerome O'Driscoll
Bridget O'Driscoll
Brian O'Riordan
Shirley Birkhahn

1959
William Aherne
Vincent Allen
Dennis Markham Buckley
Daniel Coghlan
Robert Fitzgerald
Brendan Murphy
Kathleen O'Driscoll
David O'Meara
Elizabeth Brenda O'Regan
Angela Philpott
John Power
John Noel Power

1960
Julia Rita Gould
Kornelia Kaminska
Donald Magauran
John McCarthy
Matthew Nunan
Brendan O'Gorman
Seán O'Luasa
Denis O'Mullane
Bridget O'Sullivan
Katherine Moloney
William Shalloe

1961
Peter Aherne
John Brett
Gerard Buckley
Michael Burke
Eugene Callanan
Richard Chute
John Dineen
Michael Dunne
Brian Gaule
James Kenefick
Patrick O'Brien
Stanislaus O'Flynn
Timothy O'Riordan
Michael Rekab
Joseph Stanton
Ivor Vard

1962
Hugh Barry
Thomas Callaghan
Finbarr Corkery
Mary Fitzpatrick
Edmund Heapy
John Hogan
Patrick Kidd
Patrick McDonagh
Mary Carmel Mulcahy
Seán O'Sullivan

1963
Gerry Cuddigan
Raymond Donegan
Anne Gamble
Timothy Holland
Conor O'Brien
Brian O'Callaghan
Anna Maria Jordan
John O'Connor
Fintan Quane
Kevin Quinlan
John Walsh
James Rafferty

1964
Anthony Canty
Henry Costello
Frank Daly
Gobnait Lucy
Desmond Donegan
Kathleen O'Connell
Thomas O'Neill
Ivor Rosenberg

1965
John Callanan
David Bradley
Clare Dalton
Kenneth Hall
David Heelan
Denis Keane
John Long
Timothy Mulcahy
John Murphy
William Murphy
Jeremiah O'Brien
Turlough O'Brien
Donal O'Mahony
Michael O'Meara
Peter O'Shaughnessy

1966
John Barry
Richard Dineen
Denise Flannery
Robert Gallagher
Barbara Goggin
Cornelius Murphy
John Murphy
Jeremiah Neary
Conleth O'Callaghan
Eoin O'Flynn
Brian O'Loughlin
Robert Power

1967
Timothy Brady
Thomas Brennan
Daniel Burke
Gerard Collins
Patrick Gamble
Jeremy Greene
James Hogan
Edmund Kenneally
John Kenny
Noel Mulvey
William Nunan
John O'Callaghan
Thomas O'Donovan
Charles O'Loghlin
Edward Rafferty
David Vaughan
Margaret Harty
Julia O'Regan
Elaine O'Shaughnessy
Michael Tighe

1968
Patrick Barrett
Gerald Goggin
Cornelius Madden
Myles O'Byrne
Thomas O'Donovan
Richard O'Hara
James Riordan
Jeremiah Walsh

1969
Dermot Bowles
Eileen Buckley
Denis Cramer
Thomas Cronin
Rosaleen Dinneen
Jean Dundon
Arthur Flynn
Michael Lucey
Patrick Mullane
Dorothy O'Brien
Thomas O'Brien
Thomas O'Connor
Daniel O'Donovan
Mary McCarthy
Thomas Mullins
William Ryan
Brendan Sheerin

1970
Jeremiah Collins
Patrick Daly
Denis Healy
Catherine Kilmartin
John Morley
Kenneth O'Connell
Peter Ryan
Thomas Pomeroy
Anne Whelton

1971
Charles Andrews
Michael Brodie
Michael Conway
Jeremiah Cotter
Donald Daly
Michael Devlin
Michael Keane
Eamonn Kearney
John McCarthy
William Murphy
Philip O'Connell
John O'Connor
Liam Ó'Droma
John O›Mahony
Robin O›Sullivan
John Quill
Leonard Rogers
Matthew Twomey

1972
William Anderson
Patrick Buckley
Eleanor Clifford
John Daly
Philomena Floyd
James Gleeson
Donal Goggin
Eleanor Hennessy
Catherine Keane
Mary Kelleher
David Murray
Francis O'Callaghan
John O'Connell
Cathal O'Loghlin
Niall O'Neill
Rory O'Neill
Thomas O'Sullivan
Roger Ryan
James Walsh

continued over

1973

John Collins
Maurice Fitzgerald
Patricia Fennell
Anthony Gannon
Thomas Long
Catherine McCarthy
Pauline Mitchell
Daniel Moore
James Morrison
Jerome Mullane
Gerard Murray
Thomas Nyhan
David O'Brien
Thomas O'Keeffe
Edward Quinlivan

1974

Christopher Aherne
Joseph Barry
Thomas Boland
Matthew Buckley
John Cribbin
Peter Cudmore
Martin Holohan
Michael Keane
Helen Ita Leahy
Brian Manning
Donal O'Mahony
Elizabeth Noonan
Mary O'Leary
Paul O'Toole
John Russell
Brian Twomey

1975

James Barry
Paul Callaghan
Aidan Collins
Daniel Counihan
Noel Hayes

John Kelly
Mary Kerrane
David Lehane
John Mannion
Denis Mannix
Nora Mary Murphy
Robert O'Brien
Margaret O'Driscoll
Mary O'Mahony
Alice O'Regan
William O'Rourke
William Quirke
Duncan Sleeman

1976

Patrick Casey
Monica Constant
Charles Cronin
Patrick Daly
Francis Dillon
Jeremiah Healy
Patrick Keating
Martin Kinirons
Barry Long
Francis Lucey
Mary Lucey
John Lynch
Julia McCarthy
Daniel Murphy
Denis Nagle
Francis O'Hara
Noel Ormond
Michael Ryan
Jeremiah Scannell
Peter Shorten
John Tait
James Wall
Nuala Walshe

1977

Peter Cooney
William Andrews
John Barry
Patrick Cosgrove
Ulick Cronin
Mary Clifford
Nicolas Droog
Catherine Gannon
Francis Harrington
Jeremiah Lynch
Denise MacCarthy
Denis Mangan
John McMahon
Thomas Murphy
Denis Nolan
Timothy O'Regan
Margaret O'Reilly
Michael O'Sullivan
Ursula O'Regan
Arthur Stewart
Francis Whelton

1978

Raphael Bellamy
Daniel Buckley
Michael Delaney
Daniel Fenn
David Fuller
Orla Harding
John Hogan
Cora McCarthy
Martin McDonnell
Eileen Murphy
John O'Brien
Daniel O'Connell
Cornelius O'Leary
Margaret O'Regan
Daniel O'Sullivan
Kenneth Rogers
Brendan Russell
Bemjamin Shorten
David Tuohy

BDS GRADUATES *continued*

1979
Johanna Blake
Muriel Collins
Anne Crotty
Joseph Fitzgerald
Catherine Fitzbibbon
John Goode
John Hackett
Patrick Kaar
Patrick Kelly
Anne Lynch
Niamh MacMahon
Dermot Mahony
Timothy Murphy
Ian O'Dowling
Marie O'Gorman-Kane
Eavan O'Malley Quaid
Patrick Wall

1980
Bridget Keogh
Gerard Browne
Derek Cashin
Colman Counihan
Mary Daly
Patrick Hynes
William Kiely
Michael Lane
Catherine McNamara
Patrick Morrison
Daniel O'Hanrahan
Cornelius O'Keeffe
Cornelius O'Sullivan
Geoffrey O'Sullivan
Miriam Slevin
Mary Sorensen
Berna Treacy
Helen Walsh

1981
Cyril Browne
Conor Clune
Michael Corridan
Patrick Dineen
Barbara Doyle
Patrick Donohoe
Bernice Fitzgibbon
Richard Gillman
Maurice Healy
Kevin Kenefick
Josephine Leahy
John Lee
John Lordan
Ronan Lyden
Michael Mulcahy
Thomas Mulligan
Pauline Russell
Ann O'Connor
Kevin O'Regan
William O'Sullivan
Patrick Wiseman

1982
Patrick Byrne
Eleanor Buckley
Niamh Cullinane
Daniel Cahill
Abigail Quinlan
Xavier Coleman
Eileen Crowley
Maurice Delaney
John Galvin
Finbarr Le Masney
Jeremiah Lynch
Gerard McCarthy
Joseph Mullen
Michelle Murphy
William O'Connor
Gerard O'Mahony
Gretta O'Regan
Jeremiah O'Regan

Peter O'Reilly
Gerald O'Sullivan

1983
David Casey
Catherine Corridan
Kathleen Regina Cronin
Jane Daly
Margaret Fitzgerald
Donal Fleming
Laurence Fleming
John Foley
Mary Harney
Joan Kearney
Nora Keohane
Dora Mary Kerr
Niall Le Masney
Maurice Leahy
Michael Linehan
Nora Therese Lynch
James McLoughlin
James McNamara
Matthew O'Callaghan
Rita O'Dowd
Nora Dolores O'Leary
Teresa O'Loughlin
Barry O'Regan
Patrick Power
William Reidy
Denis Ryan
Michael Shanahan

1984
Anne Jane Mary O'Connor
Anne Patricia O'Connor
Clare Canton
Brendan Coffey
Cornelius Creedon
Owen Crotty
Seamus Flynn
Roger Grufferty
Adrienne O'Halloran

continued over

Patricia Kiely
Patrick Kilker
Martin McCarthy
Michael McCarthy
Brian O'Connell
William O'Connor
Thomas Parker
Margaret Rath
Ciaran Rattigan
Asta Helleris
John Seward
Daniel Thompson
Michael O'Regan
Joanna Walsh
Maura Walsh

1985
Richard Browne
Timothy Buckley
Patrick Collins
John Cronin
Michael Cronin
Richard Fitzgerald
Helen Hassett
Finbarr Herlihy
Denis Kerrisk
Patrick Lee
Ruth Lynch
Elizabeth McStay
Liz Monahan
Paul Nolan
Noreen O'Connell
Patrick Penny
Fiona Power
Cormac Reynolds
Colm Sugrue
Nicholas Waldron
Dolores Walsh
James Walsh
Noelene Walsh

1986
Philip Christopher Barriscale
John Joseph Bowen
John Gerard Buckley
Denis Patrick Coughlan
Mary Bernadette Coveney
Patrick Gerard Creedon
Patrick Anthony Cronin
Hannah Paula Crowley
Gordon John Dalton
Dominic Joseph Patrick Finn
Miriam Susan Gibson
Mary Margaret Harding
Carol Josephine Hassett
Brian Gerard Hickey
Helena Rose Joy
Donagh Cyril Mary Kennedy
Mary Catherine Kiely
Lee Look Lan Lee Cheong
Grainne Mary McAuliffe
Alan Denis Patrick McCarthy
Robert James McStay
Aidan Martin Monahan
Brona Mary Moran
Jeremiah Patrick Mulcahy
Anastasia Elizabeth Murphy
Niall Martin Murphy
Anthony Andrew O'Connor
Joseph Francis Mary O'Connor
Margaret Mary O'Donohoe
James Martin O'Donovan
Patrick Colm O'Driscoll
Eileen Mary O'Hanlon
Donal Joseph O'Keeffe
Mary Jacqueline O'Neill
Oonagh Mary Brigid O'Regan
Denis John Regan O'Reilly
Kevin O'Rourke
Lelia Maria O'Shaughnessy
James Joseph Trant

1987
John Gerard Barry
Siobhán Mary Majella Bell
Anne Marie Brady
Gerardine Katherine Breen
Ian Gerard Broderick
Michael Gerard Brosnan
Joseph Paul Callanan
Myra Angela Clery
Eileen Mary Cronin
Lorna Maria Helen Daly
John Cyril Dermody
Margaret Valerie Donegan
Denis Francis Field
Robert Martin Gallagher
Martina Josephine Griffin
Janet Mary Heffernan
Anne Mary Hegarty
Ann Marie Hourihan
Dympna Anne Kavanagh
Norah Mary Kelleher
Kevin Christopher Kennedy
Nuala Maria King
Paul Stephen McCabe
Frances Anne O'Callaghan
Hannah Mary O'Connell
Maeve Bernadette O'Flynn
Maeve Bernadette O'Sullivan
Margaret Anne O'Sullivan
Simon Roger Pearson
Michele Blaithin Ring
Michael Gabriel Thornton

1988
Patrick Finbarr Allen
Ann Grania Barry
Thomas Gerard Bradley
Michael John Mary Crowley
Patrick Oscar Dermody
Bryan Joseph Duggan
Caroline Ann Egan

Edith Mary Finn
Kathleen Mary Fox
John Francis Furlong
Jennifer Ann Gardiner
Eavan Mary Martina Geaney
Michael Paul Hartnett
Richard Christopher Haugh
Catherine McSweeney
Rory Diarmuid Molloy
John Gerard Moriarty
Patrick Joseph O'Brien
Peter Martin Gerard O'Brien
Aidan Allan O'Dowling
Ciara Ann O'Neill
Mary Elizabeth O'Reilly
Brian Joseph O'Rourke
John Aloysius O'Sullivan
Judith Mary Phelan
Nicola Mary Judith Spillane
Paul Vivian Beirne

1989
Paul John Anthony Brady
Leo John Burke
Michael Gerard Coleman
Mary Ita Creedon
Maurice Joseph Fitzgerald
Mark Foley
Katherena Mary Galvin
Ursula Mary Gleeson
Michael Habisreutinger
Desmond Gabriel Kennedy
Fiona Margaret Mary Leahy
Lee Soo Lan Lee Cheong
Eric Pui Wai Leung
Elizabeth Ann Lyons
Fiona Elizabeth MacSweeney
Mary Ceceilia McCarthy
Seán Dominic McCarthy
John Paul Murphy
Sharon Murphy

Gerrarda Concepta O'Beirne
Finola Martina O'Connell
Colm Bartholomew O'Donovan
Michael Brian O'Leary
Anne Marie O'Neill
Ellen Geraldine O'Riordan
Maurice Gerard Quirke
Donnell Vincent Ryan
Thomas Smyth
John Michael Young

1990
Susan Maria Barry
Cornelius Finbarr Buckley
Mairéad Cashman
Paul John Conroy
Margaret Linda Corkery
Michelle Antoinette Costelloe
Timothy Michael Cronin
Dermot Jude Crowley
Niamh Noelle Crowley
Ann Deasy
Rory John Dwyer
Tomás Cian Feehely
Fiona Mary Hayes
David Jeremy Hegarty
Finbar Matthew Hillery
Aisling Mary Holland
Joseph Gilles Lecours
Diarmuid Richard Linehan
Kevin John Magee
Thomas Gerard Maher
Judith Margaret McAuley
Brian Anthony McElhinney
Bernard Daniel Murphy
Ruth Clare Murphy
Patrick Anthony O'Brien
John Michael O'Flynn
William John Patrick Ryan
Paul Finbarr Twomey

1991
Elizabeth Catherine Barrett
Thomas James Bourke
Raymond John Bradfield
John Darren Randell Broderick
Siobhán Mary Cleary
Christopher Joseph Cotter
Ann Marie Crosbie
Teresa Majella Curran
Amelia Kate Nesbitt Davis
Anna-Maria Delaney
Catherine Foley
Mary Catherine Galvin
Zita Marie Geraldine Geaney
Fiona Mary Edith Graham
Elaine Catherine Guinan
Mary Martina Hales
Blaithin Maire Hegarty
Aidan Mary Higgins
Conal Patrick Kavanagh
Joseph Anthony Kelly
Sharon Hannah Kingston
Josephine Maria Landers
June Marie Leahy
Timothy Lynch
Veronica Claire McCoy
Margaret Anne McHenry
Mary Lenora Loretto Nyhan
Matthew Joseph O'Brien
Seán Fionnbara O'Conaill
David Anthony O'Connor
Dermot Gerard O'Connor
Seighin Pol O'Diomasaigh
Padraig Cathal O'Donoghue
Aidan Philip Power
John Flannan Sheehan
Richard Mark Tobin
Enda Brendan Michael Whelan

continued over

1992

James Jeremiah Allen
Henry Vincent Brien
Patrick Brian Canty
Margaretta Marie Carr
Elizabeth Mary Cronin
John Francis Crotty
Joseph Brendan Dargan
Dolores Catherine Duffy
Stephen Patrick Finn
Jane Mary Harrington
Jo Hanna Majella Hayes
John Thomas Holland
Leandro Jimenez Carretie
Julia Bernadette Leahy
Jeremiah Anthony Linehan
Siobhán Eibhlis MacSweeney
Karl John Mangan
Brian Gerard McCabe
Niall Thomas McCarthy
Barry Richard McNicholl
Maurice Joseph Meade
Michael Finbarr O'Driscoll
Jane Mary O'Gorman
Domhnall Gerard O'Halloran
Gerard Brian O'Sullivan
Richard Anthony Tarrant
Liam Gerard Tuohy
Padraig Anthony Twomey
Helen Walsh

1993

Marie Christine Barrett
Nuala Marie Cagney
Thomas Eugene Mary Cronin
Terence Michael Crotty
Elaine Maria Dillon
Margaret Ellen Fallon
Catherine Anne Gallagher
John Francis Hennessy
Mark Patrick Hurley

Mary Hurley
Mary Anne Lee
Fiona Lyons
Brian Francis McCaughey
Kieran Liam O'Connor
Mary Eileen O'Dea
Brenda Mary O'Dowd
Timothy Joseph O'Keeffe
Ian Pierce O'Leary
Mary Bridget O'Neill
Mary Colette O'Sullivan
Paula Jane Reardon
Niall Gerard Sharkey
Derek Anthony Sheils
James Martin Tiernan
Anne Margaret Twomey
Dorcas Miriam Whitney

1994

Tomás Martin Allen
Faisal Ali Hussein Amir
Evelyn Frances Crowley
Kenneth Noel Daly
Fiona Patricia De Groot
Pauline Elizabeth Desmond
Maris Anne Maria Dillon
Margaret Claire Dunne
Ciaran Anthony Harte
Mark Arthur Joseph Henry
Joseph Hogan
Maurice Lyons
Patricia Anne Dolores McCoy
Joseph Francis Moloney
Noel David Monahan
Paul Francis Mulryan
Aidan Murphy
Mary Ha Ngeh
Sinead Maire Nic Ghearailt
Eimear Breda Mary O'Brien
Patrick Kevin O'Brien
Orla Mary O'Connor

Michael Clement O'Sullivan
Gerard Patrick Rahilly
Caillin Redican
William Mark Twomey
Caitriona Martina Walsh

1995

Al Addoomi Khaled Obaid
    Jumah Obaid
Abdul-Aziz I.H. Al Attar
Abdulaziz Abdulhai Mahadi A.
    Alshaher
Abdullah Saud Said Alsyabi
Miriam Denise Buckley
Patrick Oliver Carey
David Andrew Clancy
Thomas Joseph Corkery
Cormac Cullinane
Adrian James Dillon
Jane Patricia Godfrey
Charles Michael Haly
Patrick Joseph Noel Hartnett
Colin Hayes
Bryan Patrick Heffernan
Elaine Susan Howlett
Kevin Paul James
Michael Damian Lynagh
Niamh Joanna McCarthy
Brigid McGrath
Cormac McNamara
Edmond Andrew Murphy
Olga Ann Murphy
John Paul Newman
Mairéad Aisling Ní Shuibhne
Ruairi Padraig O'Conchubhair
Julianna Marie O'Connor
Mary Anita O'Gorman
Karen Maria O'Hanlon
Nora Marie O'Keeffe
Judith Mary O'Meara
Anne Mirriam O'Riordan

Margaret Mary O'Sullivan
Thomas Augustine Quilter
Liam Patrick Reddington
Liam Riordan
Simon Gerard Stokes
Thomas Christopher Twomey

1996
John Coleman Aherne
Nasser Mohammad
    Al-Manthery
Susan Butler
Roderick Daniel Casey
Denis Gerard Duggan
Bernadette Marie Fee
Sheila Hagan
Michelle Anne Hickey
Elizabeth Margaret Johnston
Maeve Maria Joyce
David Luke Kennedy
Bridget Rosemary Kingston
Yvonne Margaret Lonergan
Marcas Eoghan Mac
    Domhnaill
Alanna Maharaj
Marianne Agnes McHugh
John Nigel Thomas Mills
Thomas Anthony Murray
Catherine Frances O'Connor
Caroline Marian O'Doherty
Seamus O'Donnchadha
Owen Thaddeus O'Neill
Esther Mary O'Regan
Akmal Aida Othman
Eilish Maria Riordan
Mairéad Therese Riordan
Mary Martina Riordan
Denis St John Ryan
Patricia Mary Shalloe
Sandra Ann Whelan

1997
Amirham Ahmad
Salahudeen Ali Al-Bulushi
Mahmoud Abdullah Nasser
    Al-Hadrami
Bartholomew James Buckley
Maria Therese Byrne
Bridget Mary Cantwell
Lucinda Mary Carr
John Richard Stephen Chandler
Eimear Angela Cleary
Marie Elizabeth Cooke
Eric Timothy Cotter
Clodagh Carmel Crotty Ryan
Niall Patrick Shane Cummins
Denise Cunningham
Carmel Brigid Curtin
Jeremiah Patrick Daly
Elizabeth Ann Galvin
Susan Teresa Gleeson
Breeda Hennelly
Stephen James Hennessy
Nora Patricia Kearney
Elizabeth Clare Kelleher
Grainne Kieran
John Martin Linnane
Jason Christopher Long
Anthony Daniel Maher
Joseph Paul McKenna
Bridget Kathleen Murphy
Christine Anne Murphy
Clodagh Áine Ní Eocha
Margaret Ann O'Connor
Patrick James O'Connor
Paul James Gerard O'Dwyer
Triona Maire O'Flynn
Aidan Finbarr Oliver Ryan
Kathy Margaret Ryan
Colman Patrick Twomey
Robert Henry Wallace

1998
Syiral Mastura Binte Abdullah
Nawaf Faisal Al Hamer
Aisling Therese Bannon
Denis James Barry
Noelle Mary Stephanie Carey
Fionnuala Margaret Cleary
Stephen Thomas Cotter
Jeremiah John Dowling
Michael Laurence Doyle
Noorunisa Bt Shawal Hamid
Patrick Joseph Hynes
Liam Fergal Jones
Kelebogile Kgosibodiba
Maria Joan Landers
Colin John Maher
Jennifer Rachael Mountjoy
Fiona Brid Ní Chonchubhair
Gerald Michael O'Connor
Thomas Joseph O'Connor
Ronan Gerald O'Donoghue
Emily Mary O'Dwyer
Seán Toomey
Cliona Twomey

1999
Noora Khalfan Saif Al-Amri
Dalal Abdulla Al-Hakeem
Nasser Salim Obaid Al-Khaldi
Salah Abdullah Mohamed
    Al-Mandhari
Mohamed Zahran Zahir
    Al-Nabhani
Abdulaziz Hamood Hilal
    Al-Sawai
Catherine Maria Barry
Deirdre Mary Browne
Elaine Mary Browne
Michelle Elizabeth Browne
Patricia Cora Buckley

continued over

John Burke
John Joseph Shane Curtin
Muireann Rose Cush
Ronan Doyle
Grainne Maire Fleming
Thomas Noel Guinan
Freda Mary Guiney
Louise Hagan
Catherine Brigid Hallahan
Kerry Hennessy
Orla Áine Jackson
Lynda Mary Kenefick
Dervla Anne Leavy
Christopher Daniel Lynch
Ross Mac Mathuna
Jamie Maguire
Clara Maria McSwiney
Nicola Elizabeth Mulhaire
Clare Theresa Murray
Diarmuid Antaine O'Croinin
Lettice O'Leary
Anne Marie Owens
Olivia Patricia Plunkett
Peter Niall Prenter
Derek Anthony Riordan
Margaret Riordan
Bobby Segadimo
Martin Stokes

2000

Mohammed Ibrahim Al Ajami
Majda Said Al Sulaimani
Latfiya Saleem Al-Harthi
Qassim Al-Mamari
Kevin Francis Buckley
Nora Mary Curtin
Niamh Bernadette Daly
Patrice Marie Dineen
Corinne Margaret Dwyer
Cormac Finn
Ann Louise Catherine Flynn

Faith Galebole
Liam Martin Harte
Iseult Margaret Hearne
Dayangku Siti Mulyani
  Penigran Ibrahim
Norliwati Ibrahim
Karl Michael James
Aoife Mary Agnes Kelleher
Susanne Maria Rondal Kelleher
Benvon Helen Lyons
Maria Lyons
Peter Jeremiah Morrison
Grainne Siobhán Mulcare
Colm Murphy
Teresa Frances Murphy
Clodagh Marion Myers
Anna Maria Nunan
Cormac Seamus O'Coileain
Paul Gerard O'Connell
Margaret Bernice O'Connor
Michelle Therese O'Neill
Emma Catherine O'Sullivan
Martin Joseph O'Sullivan
Eithne Anne Ryan
Fiona Siobhán Ryan
Eimear Marie Toomey
Mary-Clare Elaine Tuohy
Catherine Ann Vaughan

2001

Gavin Joseph Barry
Maire Bridget Brennan
Aidan Peter Callanan
Serryth Dominic Colbert
Joanne Margaret Collins
Davina Mary Cronin
Gavin William Deasy
Marion Colette Dinan
Conor Bernard Durack
Deirdre Margaret Fahey
Michelle Mary Frost

Marina Eleanor Fuller
Fionnuala Teresa Gannon
Siobhán Maria Harnett
Bridget Marie Therese
  Harrington-Barry
Lorraine Catherine Harte
John Paul Harty
Leila Claire Kingston
Fergal Rory Philip Maguire
Niamh Joan McAuliffe
James McCormack
Margaret Mary McDonnell
Caroline O'Brien
Timothy James O'Connell
Arthur Leary O'Connor
Helen Maria O'Mullane
Patrick James Quinn
Seamus Paul Sharkey
Badiredi Tau

2002

Nadia Al-Kindy
Sinead Allis
Abdul-Hakeem Al-Masroori
Yousuf Al-Tarshi
John Thomas Patrick Bailey
Thabo Bogatsu
John Timothy Mary Browne
Niamh Mary Cashman
David John Chin Shong
Olwen Marguerite Daly
Ronan Gerard Fox
Finn Edward Geoghegan
Deirdre Eileen Hayes
Yvonne Marie Kiernan
Eadin Noelle Mary Lawless
Eilish Mary Lynch
Colm Mac Cormaic

Padraig Martin McAuliffe
Una Lisa McElroy
Keith James Murphy
Richeal Monica Ní Riordáin
Daniel Joseph O'Connor
Denis Michael O'Donovan
Josef Daniel Cahir O'Keeffe
Colm O'Loghlen
Ursula Margaret O'Mahony
Colm Seán O'Neill
Kevin Fiachra Roarty
Bairbre Ellen Stack
Mary Martina Stokes
Fiona Brid Twohig

2003
Khalid Salah Al Farsi
Naser Al-Hajeri
Ziyana Ali Al-Maskari
Torjus Ossian Baalack
Carolyn Barry Murphy
Kieran Thomas Brennan
Dominique Gabrielle Brindley
Niamh Miriam Comber
Nicholas Andrew Conway
Joanne Marguerite Costelloe
Shane Fachtna Crowley
Anthony John Curtin
Rosemarie Margaret Daly
Colin Dennison
Seoirse Gearoid Erics
Maeve Danielle Frahill
Anne Louise Gilligan
Robert Gerard Gleeson
Kathleen Margaret Harte
Audrey Margaret Hickey
Geraldine Kehoe
Julie Anna Kelleher
Grace Mary Kelly
Mary Regina Kenny
Nivash Gerard Lalloo

Farha Hanina Maidi
Tsholofelo Molefi
Michael Lawrence Mullins
Eimear Brid Murphy
James Anthony Murphy
Regina Mary Helena Murphy
Mary Catriona O'Connor
Shane Joseph O'Connor
Anne Maria O'Donnell
John Nicholas O'Mahony
Clare Oonagh Anne O'Sullivan
Robert John Philpott
Finbarr Michael Power
Andrew Frank Rowe
Kevin Patrick Ryan
Eoin Micheál Twohig
Diarmuid Pio Twomey

2004
Elaine Barry
Ciara Elaine Browne
Kathryn Marie Browne
Aidan Francis James Burke
Orla Marie Coffey
Jennifer Coughlan
Sarah Mary Ann Cusack
Patrick James John Delaney
Aileen Maria Donovan
Triona Marie Fahey
Aisling Mary Feeney
John Michael Feerick
John James Fitzpatrick
Elizabeth Mary Foad
Jennifer Marjorie Kearney
Pauraic Keogh
Eileen Maire McCarthy
Elizabeth Joanna Moloney
Patrick Francis O'Beirne
Richard John O'Brien
Owen Jeremiah Eoin O'Carroll
John Edward O'Connell

Nora Mary O'Connor
Denis Ronan O'Donovan
Carolyn O'Dwyer
Andrias Colman O'Gadhra
Susan O'Hara
Miriam Anne Quilty
Mamoon Rashid
Aman Ulhuq
William Seamus Waters
Mark Henry Wilson

2005
Maryam Said Abdullah
  Al-Araimi
Alia Al-Rahbi
Bernadette Julie Maria Barry
Niamh Ann Buckley
Eleanor Maria Burke
Maria Colette Cashman
Gillian Mary Collins
David Charles Cronin
Niall Denis Cronin
Aileen Claire Crowley
Thato Unah Entaile
Marie Joan Glavin
Michael Anthony Hayes
Anthony Nicholas James
Elaine Anne Johnston
Kenneth Patrick Keohane
Catherine Sarah Lambe
Chun Ching Liu
Kathleen Angela Lynch
Johannes Johnny Matlou
Micheál James McAuliffe
Jennifer Anne McGrath
Eoin Raymond Mills
Kefentse Charles Moatlhodi
Magdalen Mokrzanowski

continued over

Paul Patrick Michael Murphy
Victoria Anne Nason
Aoife Áine Ní Chonchubhair
Clair Joanna Nolan
Aoife O'Connor
Emer Mary O'Leary
Louise Johanna O'Leary
Caoimhe Martina O'Shea
Orla Ann Shanahan
Joseph Tidimane
Sarah Maria Tobin
Emma Ann Vahey
Niamh Walsh

2006
Miriam Louise Bourke
Mairéad Róisín Browne
Mary Grace Buckley
Paul Jonathan Patrick Canty
Helen Bernadette Cronin
Bridget Marie Fitzgerald
Rhian Fitzgerald
Jacqueline Mairéad Foley
Katie Maria Gleeson
Shauna Noelle Hannon
Michael Thomas Mark Hayes
Norette Ann Kearney
Elaine Marie Kehily
Anne Martina Kelleher
Paula Kelleher
Boitumelo Latelang
Graham Anthony McGuire
Timothy Patrick McSwiney
Shane Gabriel Mullane
Rose-Marie Mulvey
Karen Mary Murray
Marian Nagle
Mohammed Ali Al Awadi
Eoin Padraig O'Brien
Eimear Rosaleen O'Callaghan
Claire Patricia O'Connor

David Aidan O'Dowling
Kevin Daniel O'Grady
Cara Louise O'Keeffe
Cian Eric O'Meara
Rachael Maria O'Neill
Kentse Phokoje
Sarah-Kate Quinlivan
Simon Anthony Stokes

2007
Maha Al Qabendi
Kate Gemima Barry
Patricia Barry Murphy
Daniel Ronan Collins
Eileen Clodagh Collins
Mairéad Cotter
Kathryn Una Counihan
Matthew Philip Crinion
Claire Frances Curtin
Aoife Maureen Diggin
Ciara Margaret Feeney
Jacqueline Michelle Harnett
Emmett Thomas Hegarty
Chililo Botho Jorosi
Justin Michael Kearney
Raymond Patrick Kelleher
Basil Desmond Kelly
Siobhán Mary Lucey
Diarmuid Moloney
Bairbre Mary O'Donoghue
Morgan Paul O'Gara
Donnchadh O'Morain
Marie Nano O'Neill
Maeve Julie O'Sullivan
Danielle Ellen Marie Quinlivan
Ofentse Daniel Raditaolana
Elizabeth Anne Ryan
Jason Singh
Evelyn Maria Tobin

2008
Yacoub Al Shammari
Maryam Abdullah Al-Kandari
Fatima Al-Sarraf
Hussain Al-Wazzan
Darryl Jonathan Barry
Gregg Barry
Barbara Patricia Carey
Elaine Josepha Maria Casey
Anita Teresa Colman
Jennifer Frances Monica Cotter
Claragh Jane Drake
Aoife Maura Farrell
Nora Sybil Hopkins
Eamon Howard Bowles
Laura Anne Kirwan
Eoin Francis Lehane
Cindy Maharaj
Laura Ann McGrath
Edel Marie Moloney
Shane Gerard Mulchrone
Sinead Marita Murray
Susan Nagle
Noirín Áine Ní Chiosain
Ciara Elizabeth Ní Chonaill
Grania Catherine O'Connell
Kate Mary O'Keeffe
Killian Martin Francis Power
Nicholas Quong Sing
Monica Jane Ryan
Moo Keun Sung
Stephen James Tangney
Mphoentle Thangwane
Mary Elizabeth Turnbull
Bernard Timothy Twomey
Jennifer Mary Waldron
Fergal Joseph Walsh
Mary Clare Walsh

2009

Mohammad Al Fahim
Hesham Ali
John Bresnan
Alice Margaret Cleary
Alison Jane Comerford
Michelle Catherine Connolly
Susan Marie Crean
Barry William Crowley
Carol Agnes Dineen
Wafa Hayat
Ellen Margaret Healy
Micheál James Healy
Claire Marie Hevican
Eimear Anne Hurley
Ronan John Kavanagh
Mary Catherine Kearney
Paul Gerrard Charles Kielty
Dennis Semlan Lee Chong
Sondos Madi
Unoziba Makocha
Caroline McCarthy
David Michael McGoldrick
Ahmad Merza
Eric Mokgweetsi
Norrie June Moloney
Sarah Louise Morrissey
Geraldine Patricia Murray
Laura Maria O'Sullivan
Kabo Onkemetse Phillips
Graham Christopher Quilligan
Ian Michael Reynolds
Seamus Michael Ryan
Amel Sami
Mary Patricia Ward
Faizan Zaheer

2010

Nurul Iza Adnan
Mohamed Al Jneibi
Aoife Áine Bambury
Elizabeth Calnan Boland
Erin Cecelia Bolton
Marian Cottrell
Fionnuala Cowhie
Julie Anne Cronin
Sarah Mary Delap
Martha Dempsey
Michael Patrick Durkan
Cathal Patrick Hayes
Ontiretse Kebalepile
Wyatt Lintott
Jean Paula Long
Julia Therese Mangan
Sarah Jane Mannion
Una Maire McAuliffe
Daisy Eileen McCarthy
Leone Marian McCarthy
Elizabeth Mary Murphy
Lorna Anna Murphy
Ciara Marie Noonan
Joseph Bonang Nyepetsi
Stephen Daniel O'Connor
Orla Maire O'Herlihy
Cathy O'Leary
Finbar Anthony O'Mahony
Ronan David O'Neill
Kopano Ramotlabaki
Ruth Mary Scanlon
Emma Mary Sheehan
Sebastian Sehinson
Harry Lightfoot Stevenson
Richard Joseph Stokes
Han Jin Suk
Khumo Tlhalerwa
Claire Brigid Waldron

2011

Hessah Al Jiran
Patrick Barry
Louise Mary Canny
Claire Denise Costelloe
Irene Ann Cullinane
David Noel Finnegan
Martin Gerard Forde
Eliana Hadjiantonis
Joseph Flynn Hanley
Stephanie Mary Healy
Kate Jacinta Horgan
Helen Marie Lane
Lee Sa Lim
Cian Joseph Lowney
Katherine Ruth McCarthy
Sarah Jane McGuckian
Amanda Louise McLaughlin
Tiyapo Motsamai
Ailbhe Louise Murphy
Eamon Daniel Nugent
Eibhlin O'Donoghue
Sinead Mairéad O'Dwyer
Fiona Eileen O'Leary
Laura Anita O'Sullivan
Moubarak Othman Othman
Jennifer Mary Owens
Jay Patel
Paul Ryan
Niamh Maire Scanlon
Mary Sheehan
Tsing Wein Tan

continued over

2012

Catherine Mary Ahern
Ahmed A H A H Alsarraf
Peter Stephen Clune
Fiona Veronica Counihan
Alma Creaven
Graham Benjamin Morton
  Deane
Ann Marie Martha Downey
James Flood
Claire Noreen Foley
Tshepo Frank
Muhammad Kamil Hassan
Eimear Catriona Herlihy
Kabelo Kefhilwe
Caitriona Johanna Kennelly
Kathleen Mary McCarthy
Sally Bridget McCarthy
Ghadeer Mohammad
Mahfaruddin Mohammed
Nadzirah Mohammed Suffian
Kago Moshoeshoe
Barry Peter Mulrean
Jill Mary O'Donnell
Shane O'Dowling-Keane
Aoife Maire O'Dwyer
Caroline O'Dwyer
Leah Doreen O'Halloran
Eileen Margaret O'Mahony
Rozelle Lynne Owens
Julia Norah Quinlan
Marie Alana Sanfey
Tiroyaone Semumu
Jane Margaret Stack
Neil Tully
Jo Lin Wong
Ivan Woulfe

2013

Nik Nur Syazwani Ahmad
  Radzi
Kawthar Al-Ali
Áine Therese Barry
Hayley Brahm
Tanya Chacko
Xin Yi Michele Chia
Niamh Coffey
Frances Connors
Ciara Gabrielle Ennis
Gavin John Fitzgerald
Aileen Marie Foley
Emma Mary Franks
Michelle Ellen Fung
Michael Joseph Griffin
Emily Mary Higgins
Erica Pey Wen Hii
Maeve Áine Kenefick
Mpho Kgosi
Christopher Legare
Keamogetse Magudu
Nadine Maire McCarthy
David William McGibney
Michelle McSweeney
Ratang Moratiwa Mokgosi
Marguerite Moloney
Ian Finbar Mulvey
Thomas Augustine Murphy
Orna Doireann Ni Choileain
Hanis Nor Nasarudin
Gavin John Nugent
Áine Treise O'Herlihy
Kaelan Joseph O'Shea
Bonolo Blessed Odirile
Brendan Anthony Quinn
Dikabelo Ratshipa

Christopher James Ryan
Siti Nadia Saleh
John Bernard Spillane
Aoife Brid Stack
Simon Mervyn Sweetnam
Tun Nur Syahirah Tun Razak
Lucy Walsh
Orla Marie Walsh

Ph.D. GRADUATES

Denis O'Mullane, 1971
Louis Buckley, 1978
Gerard Buckley, 1979
John Joseph Clarkson, 1987
Helen Pauline Whelton, 1989
Roger Philip Ellwood, 1993
Dympna Anne Kavanagh, 1994
Peter Edward Hayden, 1995
Judith Ann Cochran, 1999
Ayyaz Ali Khan, 2001
Paul Vivian Beirne, 2003
Khalid Al-Kindy, 2004
Gerard Noel Woods, 2005
Eleanor Maria Ann O'Sullivan, 2006
Deirdre Mary Browne, 2008
Nada Mirghani Sanhouri, 2010
Edel Margaret Flannery, 2010
Richeal Monica Ní Riordáin, 2011
Nadia Khalifa, 2011
Lamyia M. Anweigi, 2012
Gerald John McKenna, 2013
Jeremiah Liam Lynch, 2013

MASTERS DENTAL PUBLIC HEALTH

Paul Vivian Beirne, 1999
Mary Margaret Boyce, 1999
Riana Mary Clarke, 1999
Joseph Green, 1999
Mary Helena Haran, 1999
Michael Gerard Shanahan, 1999
Helen Pauline Whelton, 1999
Stephen Peter Brightman, 2000
David John Clarke, 2000
Nader Farvardin, 2000
Mary Antoinette Nolan, 2000
Elizabeth Julia Noonan, 2000
Thomas Aloysius Nyhan, 2000
Mary Gorretti O Connor, 2000
Catriona Maire Majella Roe, 2000
Mary Bridget Tuohy, 2000
Adrianne Brigid Dolan, 2001
Mary Margaret Antoinette Harding, 2001
Michael Gerard Mulcahy, 2001
Mary Teresa Agnes Coleman, 2002
Michael Anthony Donaldson, 2002
Ruth Emily Gray, 2002
David Anthony O Connor, 2002
Susan Teresa Gleeson, 2004
Ann Carmel McKeon, 2004
Isam Mohamed Ahmed Idris, 2004
Siobhan Maeve Coakley, 2007
Catherine Martina Donnelly, 2007
Elizabeth Margaret Dunne, 2007
Mary Louisa Gormley, 2007
Jeremiah Liam Lynch, 2007
Margaret Mary Josephine McDonnell, 2007
James Joseph Paul Mullen, 2007
Makiko Nishi, 2007
Patrick James Quinn, 2007
Anne Marie Crotty, 2011
James Flahavan, 2011
Mutahira Waqar Ahmed Lone, 2011
Syed Muhammad Misbahuddin, 2011
Eimear Brid Murphy, 2011
Finola Martina O Connell, 2011
Kudirat Jimoh, 2013

DENTAL HYGIENISTS, 1995–2013

1995
Mary Martina Anne Holohan
Karen Antoinette Lehane
Elizabeth Susan Mahony
Zita Josephine White

1996
Sheila Mary Buckley
Jean Marie Carson
Rosaleen Sharon Tina Clarke
Gail Farrell
Lucita Helen Mary Fenton
Bernardine Maria O'Donovan

1997
Margaret Louise Bourke
Julie Anne Flynn
Caroline Glynn
Norah Majella Murray
Catherine Anne Rhattigan

1998
Paula Tracy Carroll
Patricia Audrey Corkery
Catherine Theresa Ann Hagan
Jillian Ann Murphy
Arran Slavin
Catherena Sweeney

1999
Margaret Annette Crisham
Linda Mary Norah Feehan
Mary Claire Flood
Caroline Helena Horgan
Aoife Christine Mary Kelly
Moira Patricia McGovern
Margaret O'Brien
Maire Gobnait O'Callaghan

2000
Niamh Theresa Collins
Mary Sorcha Cronin
Loretta Mary Jordan
Clare Josephine McGovern
Gillian Clare Murphy
Jacqueline Murphy
Jennifer Anne O'Keeffe
Ann Maria Ryan
Julianne Ryan
Grace Philomena Young

2001
Laura Sinead Bowles
Anne Marie Martina Brady
Ann Geraldine Conway
Christina Cronin
Yolande Keane
Amy Ruth Kelly
Deirdre Marie Leonard
Mary Bridget Looby
Marian Ann Moran
Lynn Maria Moynihan
Patricia Mary O'Connor
Aisling Maria O'Leary
Muire Brid Sweeney
Vanessa Dawn West

2002
Bernadette Grace Ruth Buckley
Lia Mary Coppinger
Ciara Ann Creamer
Teresa Regina Doyle
Siobhán Marie Duffy
Claire Bridget Fahy
Grainne Antoinette Farrell
Paula Mary Lyons
Paula Macken
Bridget Caitriona Murphy
Eithne O'Neill
Louise Jacqueline Strutt
Marcella Tuite
Vera Breege Ward

2003
Elaine Mary Theresa Cannon
Elizabeth Marie Cremin
Lorraine Margaret Doyle
Mary Majella Harrington
Geraldine Heffernan
Julie Karen Kearney
Selena Louise Leonard
Deidre Margaret McGerty
Rosaleen McPadden
Róisín Anne Moloney
Colette Mary Nix
Carol Mary O'Brien

2004

Sinead Marie Beattie
Michelle Marie Burns
Refellia Donovan
Theresa Jude Dunne
Sharon Marie Fennell
Elena Loreley Hopwood
Caroline Jean Keating
Isobell Mary Keyes
Brona Stephanie McDaniel
Sharon Rose McLoughlin
Brenda Margaret O'Connell
Kellie Ann O'Shaughnessy
Marie Geraldine Reddington
Manjit Kaur Sandhu
Martina Staunton
Teresa Mary Walsh

2005

Mairéad Olive Buckley
Sheila Noelle Conroy
Anne Elizabeth Corry
Sharon Patricia Cotter
Siobhán Caitlin Gargan
Nadine Hoey
Esmarie Husemeyer
Ann Marie Mollaghan
Eilish Mary Ryan
Niamh Catherine Ryan

2006

Catherine Mary Ahern
Carol Majella Bergin
Sarah Anne Carbery
Aisling Patricia Conneely
Rosario Monica Martha
    Costello
Ciara Concepta Finlay
Ailbhe Mary Healy
Vera Sarah Eileen Hutchinson
Lorraine Anne Kelly
Paula Catherine Lowry
Róisín Sinead Moran
Sheila Carmel Murphy
Siobhán O'Neill
Mia Anushka Radovanovich

2007

Eileen Catherine Allen
Paula Mary Cavanagh
Nora Yvonne Coleman
Neill Thomas Cullen
Caroline Daly
Susan Lawlor
Marguerite Helena Lyons
Niamh Susanne McMahon
Ciara Kathleen Meyler
Leonora Mary Moran
Imelda Margaret Shanahan
Elizabeth Walsh
Amanda Louise Walton
Carol Cleary

2008

Clare Patricia Craughwell
Emer Colette Doody
Frances Alexander Downey
Rebecca Hinds
Eimear Anne King
Martha Lynch
Jennifer Ann Mellerick
Fiona Josephine Murray
Judith O'Dwyer
Lorraine Gillian O'Halloran
Emma Jane Ryan
Jennifer Eileen Shanahan
Pearl Angela Veale

2009

Elaine Bannon
Susan Angela Barrett
Eimear Maria Casey
Karen Mary Comerford
Carol Patricia Downey
Martina Ann Gallagher
Michelle Therese Lyne
Amie Jane McManus
Joelle Patricia Mary Mousset
Frances Quinn
Gemma Majella Ryan
Elaine Ann Walsh

continued over

2010

Caroline Marie Coen
Christine Mary Dorgan
Grainne Helena Johnson
Mairéad Noelle McLoughlin
Andrea Marie Murray-Lambert
Lynsey Lorraine Neill
Claire Teresa O'Connor
Annemarie Patricia O'Rourke
Mary Rosario Owens
Caroline Prendergast
Aisling Veronica Reynolds
Michelle Linda Sheehan
Angela Margaret Tierney
Aoife Marie Burke

2011

Elizabeth Mary Byrne
Nora Christine Clifford
Emma Jane Cosgrove
Aisling Mary Counihan
Ciara Marie Drummond
Donna Dunleavy
Kate Ferron
Anita Nora Horgan
Sharon Louise Kenny
Denise Mary Looby
Helen Marguerite Loomes
Louise Mary Meehan
Claire Alice O'Sullivan

2012

Amanda Arigho
Anne-Marie Brennan
Elena Commins
Katie French
Sharon Gaughan
Lisa Hennessy
Claire Kennelly
Cynthia Knox
Aoife Lawlor
Julianne Lowry
Alma McNally
Rachel Noonan
Tina O'Shea
Yvonne Walsh

2013

Rachel Cafferkey
Michelle Cotter
Mary Dennehy (Madden)
Anna Rose Drumm
Ann Marie Flannery
Clodagh French
Salina Heaney
Noelle Kelly
Ciara Mullins
Louise Nugent
Christine O'Callaghan
Jennifer O'Riordan
Gillian Shannon
Siobhán Walsh

DENTAL NURSES, 2004–11

Anne-Marie Brennan, 2004
Olivia Buttimer, 2004
Annette Cahill, 2004
Lara Coffey, 2004
Marie Cooney, 2004
Aisling Dee, 2004
Deirdre Donnelly, 2004
Elaine Dowling, 2004
Deirdre Dunne, 2004
Martine Greenlee, 2004
Lorraine Hadnett, 2004
Valerie Hillgrove, 2004
Hilary Harrington, 2004
Tara Jennings, 2004
Breda Kelleher, 2004
Nevenka Klemencic, 2004
Emily Lane O'Neill, 2004
Orla Leahy, 2004
Lisa Linane, 2004
Yvonne McCarthy, 2004
Ciara Meyler, 2004
Helen Mills, 2004
Grace Murphy, 2004
Valerie Murphy, 2004
Ciara O'Brien, 2004
Elaine O'Bryne, 2004
Susan O'Donoghue, 2004
Laura O'Donovan, 2004
Jill O'Donnell, 2004
Gemma O'Leary, 2004
Paula O'Neill, 2004
Maria O'Sullivan, 2004
Yvonne O'Sullivan, 2004
Joanne Quiorke, 2004
Denise Renehan, 2004
Jennifer Shanahan, 2004
Amanda Walton, 2004
Marie Cooney, 2004
Collette Barry, 2005
Norita Brosnan, 2005
Marie Carey, 2005

Miriam Casey, 2005
Sharon Cooney, 2005
Grace Corcoran, 2005
Kathy Cotter, 2005
Michelle Cowan, 2005
Audrey Dempsey, 2005
Michelle Doherty, 2005
Teresa Fitzgerald, 2005
Aisling Fitzsimons, 2005
Leona Foley, 2005
June Grant, 2005
AnneMarie Healy, 2005
Anita Horgan, 2005
Tara Kearney, 2005
Maire Kennedy, 2005
Emily Lane-O'Neill, 2005
Aislinn Lehane, 2005
Juliane Lowry, 2005
Sarah Lucey, 2005
Sally Mynard, 2005
Nicola McCarthy, 2005
Breffni Murray, 2005
Jolita Navikaite, 2005
Emma O'Brien, 2005
Ciara O'Connell, 2005
Loretta O'Connell, 2005
Laura O'Dwyer, 2005
Catherine O'Flaherty, 2005
Lorraine O'Mahoney, 2005
Ruth O'Mahony, 2005
Amy O'Neill, 2005
Annmarie O'Rourke, 2005
Tina Ryan, 2005
Elizabeth Spillane, 2005
Miriam Tuttle, 2005
Tracey Byrne-Doyle, 2006
Colette Costello, 2006
Marie Johnson, 2006
Deborah Kelleher, 2006
Mairéad Malone, 2006
Christine O'Callaghan, 2006

Meadbh Devane, 2006
Michelle O'Connor, 2006
Helena O'Riordan, 2006
Orla O'Sullivan, 2006
Amanda Arigho, 2006
Claudine Ashe, 2006
Avril Bardsley, 2006
Jane Benson, 2006
Collette Buckley, 2006
Eimear Buckley, 2006
Amanda Cambridge, 2006
Aoibhinn Corcoran, 2006
Roberta Daly, 2006
Sandra Daly, 2006
Mary Duggan, 2006
Fiona Fitzgerald, 2006
Tanya Grainger, 2006
Emily Hagan, 2006
Fay Kellett, 2006
Andrea Keohane, 2006
Claudia Kiely, 2006
Ciara Lordan, 2006
Carmel Lynch, 2006
Rita McCarthy, 2006
Marie Neville, 2006
Carol O'Leary, 2006
Elaine O'Shea, 2006
Orla O'Callaghan, 2006
Victoria O'Doherty, 2006
Siobhán O'Sullivan, 2006
Jessica Rojas, 2006
Tracey Allen, 2007
Lisa Brosnan, 2007
Juliet Carroll, 2007
Lorraine Coulter, 2007
Clare Justine Daly, 2007
Vanessa De Vere, 2007
Sinead Deasy, 2007
Teresa Dempsey, 2007
Terri Donovan, 2007
Evelyn Golden, 2007

continued over

Sarah Guiney, 2007
Vanessa Hallahan, 2007
Karen Hennessy, 2007
Elaine Kearney, 2007
Sabrina Kelly, 2007
Davina Kelly, 2007
Kate Kisinska, 2007
Deirdre Leslie, 2007
Tuuli Linder, 2007
Mary Madden, 2007
Orla McLaughlin, 2007
Ciara Nolan, 2007
Siobhán O'Callaghan, 2007
Jilly O'Connor, 2007
Siobhán O'Mahony, 2007
Jennifer O'Riordan, 2007
Shirley Ryan, 2007
Jenna Wade, 2007
Debbie Walsh, 2007
Iryna Belaya, 2007
Siobhán Cooley, 2007
Eimear Cooney, 2007
Rosemarie Hearne, 2007
Louise Kiely, 2007
Pamela Costello, 2007
Lorraine Coughlan, 2007
Fiona Enright, 2007
Bridget Fitzgerald, 2007
Marguerite Lanigan, 2007
Carmel O'Brien, 2007
Geraldine Quinn, 2007
Paula Bergin, 2008
Sonya Marie Cronin, 2008
Linda Dennehy, 2008
Sharon Eaton, 2008
Lydia Farrell, 2008
Lorraine Fehily, 2008
Katie Halligan, 2008
Orla Murdock, 2008
Natalie Murray, 2008
Rachel Noonan, 2008

Elaine Nyhan, 2008
Elaine O'Callaghan, 2008
Siobhán O'Leary, 2008
Alicia O'Driscoll, 2008
Laura O'Sullivan, 2008
Alena Pesavova, 2008
Jennifer Russell, 2008
Caitriona Ryan, 2008
Elaine Taggart, 2008
Nicola Barry, 2008
Róisín Cooney, 2008
Jayne Merrigan, 2008
Jennifer Murphy, 2008
Celia O'Connor, 2008
Deirdre Whitty, 2008
Helen Angley, 2008
Caroline Crean, 2008
Paula Dalton, 2008
Jean Delahunty, 2008
Kathryn Fahy, 2008
Anne Gleeson, 2008
Paula Hennessy Carroll, 2008
Ann-Marie Judge, 2008
Claire Kelly, 2008
Aoife Kilmartin, 2008
Ciara Long, 2008
Olga Tkacova, 2008
Lisa Vaughan, 2008
Paula Baker Guerineau, 2008
Susan Lynch, 2008
Patricia Moloney, 2008
Tina O'Shea, 2008
Elaine Kearney, 2008
Ciara Nolan, 2008
Jilly O'Connor, 2008
Eimear Cooney, 2008
Bridget Fitzgerald, 2008
Gillian Brazier, 2009
Joanne Cody, 2009
Tina Coffey, 2009
Jenika Cox, 2009

Julie Daly, 2009
Pauline Daly, 2009
Amy Dempsey, 2009
Amanda Doyle, 2009
Lydia Farrell, 2009
Siobhán Fennell, 2009
Helen Fitzgibbon, 2009
Leona Fogg, 2009
Bernie Gahon, 2009
Katarzyna Gorecka, 2009
Sarah Hosey, 2009
Rachel Humphreys, 2009
Debbie Magee, 2009
Regina McSweeney, 2009
Monica Mera, 2009
Katy Moore, 2009
Orla Murphy, 2009
Kate Nagle, 2009
Marta Niechwiadowicz, 2009
Alice O'Connor, 2009
Adele O'Keeffe, 2009
Elaine O'Shea, 2009
Agne Pinkeviciute, 2009
Caroline Ryan, 2009
Anne Marie Scully, 2009
Natalie Baldwin, 2009
Antoinette Behan, 2009
Kelly Brennan, 2009
Janet Browne, 2009
Eimear Cooney, 2009
Fiona Cullen, 2009
Sarah-Louise Dreelan, 2009
Sharon Holden, 2009
Elena Hutanu, 2009
Marianne Jackman, 2009
Ewelina Klek, 2009
Rosaleen Lonergan, 2009
Aoife Maher, 2009
Orla Manahan, 2009
Kelly Anne O'Leary, 2009
Emma Jane Woods, 2009

Bernie Arthur Flynn, 2009
Gillian Browne, 2009
Edel Greaney, 2009
Paula Hennessy Carroll, 2009
Lenka Jurgosova, 2009
Gemma Keane, 2009
Aimee Lamb, 2009
Caroline Lynch, 2009
Shinead McMahon, 2009
Carol Naughton, 2009
Anne O'Sullivan, 2009
Erika Schimf, 2009
Mairéad Shanahan, 2009
Hazel Anderson, 2010
Kellie Blake, 2010
Laura Buckley, 2010
Deborah Buckley, 2010
Evelyn Curtin, 2010
Debbie Magee, 2010
Denise Foley, 2010
Leigh Johnston, 2010
Katarzyna Kurgan, 2010
Claire Lester, 2010
Evelyn Llewellyn, 2010
Sarah Lucey, 2010
Mairéad Malone, 2010
Deirdre McGrath, 2010
Ciara Moloney, 2010
Tara Murphy, 2010
Denise O'Leary, 2010

Eleanor Noelle O'Leary, 2010
Aoife O'Mahony, 2010
Michelle Seward, 2010
Elaine Sheehan, 2010
Jenny Slattery, 2010
Orla Spillane, 2010
Michelle Stone, 2010
Ellen Wharton, 2010
Annita Cahill, 2010
Patrice Cummins, 2010
Joanne Dalton, 2010
Emma Harty, 2010
Elena Hutanu, 2010
Marie Kelly, 2010
Brita McCartan, 2010
Antoinette O'Gorman, 2010
Catherine Clifford, 2010
Megan Coughlan, 2010
Caitriona Cullinan, 2010
Niamh Fitzgerald, 2010
Elaine Madden, 2010
Orla Madigan, 2010
Áine McKenna, 2010
Grainne O'Toole, 2010
Gillian Shannon, 2010
Kelly-Ann Young, 2010
Alayne Margaret Berkery, 2011
Aoife Breen, 2011
Alma Clohessy, 2011
Michelle Connolly, 2011

Emer Coughlan, 2011
Louise Coughlan, 2011
Margaret Cosgrave, 2011
Ruth Delaney, 2011
Charlotte Downing, 2011
Isabel Mary Fenton, 2011
Joanne Foley, 2011
Marie Fuller, 2011
Jacinta Healy, 2011
Ciara Hendy, 2011
Olivia Hickey, 2011
Jennifer Marie Kiely, 2011
Gloria Linehan, 2011
Denise Lordan, 2011
Kate McCarthy, 2011
Emma Murphy, 2011
Ciara O'Brien, 2011
Yvonne O'Connell, 2011
Laura O'Donnell, 2011
Celine O'Flynn, 2011
Jennifer O'Mahony, 2011
Aoife O'Sullivan, 2011
Claire Palmer, 2011
Chloe Marie Sheehan, 2011
Amy Stuart, 2011
Susan Mary Toner, 2011
Linda Wharton, 2011
Fiona Kelly, 2011
Lynsey Phelan, 2011
Melissa Warring, 2011

DENTAL TECHNICIANS

1983/84

Denis Brennan
John Sommers
William Sheridan
Rory O'Connor
Joseph McNamara
Patrick McGoldrick
Thomas Cooper
John Buckley

1984/85

Gregory Coleman
Patrick Small
Karol Reidy
Mary McEniff
Kieran O'Callaghan
Helen Fleming

1985/86

Maria Hickey
Edward O'Mahony
Patrick Langton
Colum Sower
Barry Barne
John McCormack
Paul Benson
David Noonan

1986/87

Catherine Cooper
Pater Kaak
David Leahy
Michael McGeown
Frank O'Donovan
Irene Reed

1988/89

Not available.

1989/90

Susan O'Connor
Mary Scally
Hugh Swan

NOTED STAFF & ALUMNI

Deans of CUDSH
Hubert O'Keeffe
George Sheedy
William Perihco
Israel Scher
Jack Daunt
Barry Collins
Gordon Russell
Brian Barrett
Louis Buckley
Denis O'Mullane
Robbie McConnell
Finbarr Allen
Martin Kinirons

Deans of the Faculty of Dentistry, Royal College of Surgeons Ireland
Norman Butler
Brian Barrett
Tim Holland
P.J. Byrne

Presidents of the Dental Council
Martin Holohan
Joe Lemasney

Presidents of the International Association for Dental Research
Helen Whelton
John Clarkston

Presidents of the Irish Dental Association
E. Sheldon Friel
Jack Daunt
Jim O'Meara
Barry Collins
George McSweeney
Chris Collins
Norman Butler
Jerry Healy
Noel Power
Noel Walsh
Joe Lemasney
Martin Holohan
John Barry

Members of UCC Governing Body
Denis O'Mullane
Helen Whelton

TEACHING & LEARNING IN HIGHER EDUCATION POSTGRADUATES

Certificates

2005
Edith Allen
Christine McCreary
Eleanor O'Sullivan
Helen Whelton

2007
John Brown
Frank Burke
Catherine Gorman
Patricia McDermott

2008
Martina Collins
Mary Harrington
Anne Holohan
Claire Murphy
Siobhán Murray
Anne O'Keeffe
Noel Ray

2009
Maire Kelly
Richeal Ní Riordáin
Mary O'Reilly

2010
Sharon Curtin
Caroline Horgan
Fiona MacSweeney
Gerald McKenna
Siobhán McSweeney
Derry Mulcahy
Christopher Stewart
Hassan Ziada

2012
Elizabeth Kelleher
Pamela Binks
Helena Guinea
Eimear Hurley
Helen Nwokoye

2013
Paul Brady
Martina Hayes
Michael McAuliffe
Antonios Theocharopoulos
Emma Warren

Masters Degrees

2007
Eleanor O'Sullivan

2010
Anne Holohan
Claire Murphy
Siobhán Murray
Anne O'Keeffe
Mary Harrington

2012
Siobhán McSweeney

Diplomas

2006
Edith Allen
Christine McCreary
Eleanor O'Sullivan
Helen Whelton

2008
Frank Burke
Catherine Gorman

2009
Martina Collins
Mary Harrington
Anne Holohan
Claire Murphy
Siobhain Murray
Anne O'Keeffe

2010
Mary O'Reilly

2011
Sharon Curtin
Caroline Horgan
Mary Kelly
Fiona MacSweeney
Gerald McKenna
Siobhán McSweeney
Richeal Ní Riordáin

2012
Hassan Ziada

2013
Pamela Binks
Eimear Hurley
Elizabeth Kelleher
Helen Nwokoye

2013 CORK DENTAL SCHOOL & HOSPITAL STAFF

Consultants

Finbarr Allen	Restorative
Frank Burke	Restorative
Denis Field	Orthodontics
Martin Kinirons	Dean of School & Hospital
Robert McConnell	Restorative
Christine McCreary	Oral Medicine
Donal McDonnell	Dental Radiology
Declan Millett	Orthodontics
Duncan Sleeman	Oral Surgery
Hassan Ziada	Restorative
Chris Cotter	Oral Surgery

College Lecturers/Specialists

Edith Allen	Restorative
Catherine Gallagher	Oral Surgery
Patricia McDermott	Orthodontics
Noel Ray	Restorative
Chris Stewart	Oral Health & Development

Professors

Finbarr Allen
Martin Kinirons
Robert McConnell
Duncan Sleaman
Helen Whelton

Lecturer in Dental Technology

Antonios Theocharopoulos	Restorative

Lecturer in Dental Technology (Orthodontics)

John Brown	Orthodontics

Part-time Lecturer in Conscious Sedation

Paul Brady	Oral Surgery

Lecturer in Medical Healthcare Ethics

Kieran Doran	School of Medicine

Part-time Lecturer

Eleanor O'Sullivan	Oral Surgery

continued over

Senior Instructor Dental Technician

Joe Hallissey   Restorative

Lecturer in Behavioural Science

Sharon Curtin

Administration

Jane Ahern	Switchboard
Elizabeth Cronin O'Flynn	Restorative Lab Invoices
Terry Cullinane	PA to Prof Kiniorns
Ann Marie Doran	Restorative
Anne Dunlea	Supervisor Receptions
Elizabeth Flynn	Research
Helena Guiney	Research
Deirdre Healy	Reception Postgrad Ortho
Carol Horan	Human Resource Manager
Philomena Johnson	Reception
Mary Keelan	PA to Dean of School & Hosp.
Eamonn Kiely	Facilities Manager
Ann Marie Leahy	PA to Prof. Millett
Jenny Barnett	Manager
Lisa Morgan	Restorative
Michael Murphy	Finance Manager
Neil Nash	IT Administrator
Catherine Nevin	CPD Coordinator
Bernadette O'Donoghue	Reception
Claire O'Keeffe	PA to the Manager
Paula Rose	Reception
Bernadette Sweeney	Switchboard
Helen Tyrell	PA Dr Gallagher
Mary Wade	Dental School Office

3D Imaging Technical Assistant

Niamh Kelly   *Postgraduate Ortho*

NCHD

Paul Brady	*Clinical Fellow*	Oral Surgery
Eimear Hurley	*Clinical Fellow*	Paediatric
Martina Kelleher	*Clinical Fellow*	Restorative
Elaine Marie Kehily	*Senior House Officer*	Oral Surgery
Gerry McKenna	*Clinical Fellow*	Restorative
Kevin Mellan	*Registar*	Restorative

Postgraduate Orthdontics Students

Siobhán McMorrow
Lamis Koshak
Inam Heulfe
Erfan Salloum

Part-time Clinical Teaching Staff

Deirdre Browne	Paediatric	
Michael Crowley	Restorative	
Peter Cudmore	Paediatric	
John Foley	Restorative	
Liam Harte	Oral Surgery	
Aileen Hayes	Paediatric	
Martin Holohan	Restorative	
Elizabeth Kelleher	Restorative	
Nuala Lyden	Restorative	
Barry Lynch	Restorative	*Career break*
Fiona MacSweeney	Restorative	
Joseph McKenna	Oral Surgery	
Tom McCarthy	Oral Surgery	
Mary McConnell	Restorative	
Siobhán McSweeney	Restorative	
Aidan Monahan	Restorative	
Derek Mulcahy	Restorative	
Donal O'Keeffe	Oral Surgery	
Mary O'Reilly	Restorative	
Eleanor O'Sullivan	Oral Surgery	
Billy Waters	Oral Surgery	

continued over

Nursing

Noeleen Coomey	*RGN*	DOPD
Eileen Foley	*Clinical Nurse Manager*	DOPD
Teresa Grogan	*RGN*	DOPD
Catherine Hegarty	*Clinical Nurse Manager*	
Leona Kelleher	*RGN*	DOPD
Maire Kelly	*Clinical Nurse Manager*	
Catherine Kingston	*RGN*	DOPD
Eileen Leonard	*RGN*	DOPD
Mary McCarthy	*RGN*	Oral Surgery
Mary Moloney	*Acting Dir. of Nursing*	
Katherine Morrissey Moran	*RGN*	CSSD
Gemma Napier	*RGN*	DOPD
Delores O'Brien		DOPD
Nora O'Mahony	*RGN*	Oral Surgery
Janice Sweeney	*RGN*	DOPD
Ann Stritch	*RGN*	DOPD
Toni Whelan	*RGN*	DOPD

Dental Nurses

Pamela Binks	Joan McDermott
Patricia Bourke	Colette Murray
Gillian Bradley	Norma Murray
Jacqueline Bray	Jennifer Newman
Veronica Burton	Fiona O'Callaghan
Louise Carmody	Muriel O'Connor
Sheila Casey	Grainne O'Donovan
Jacinta Collins (DOPD)	Emer O'Dwyer
Catherine Cronin	Deirdre O'Shea
Robeta Daly	Mary M. O'Sullivan
Vanessa De Vere (*research nurse*)	Judith Riordan
Maria Doolan	Philomena Scannell
Nellie Healy	Amelia Spillane
Sinead Lane	Elizabeth Thompson
Renie Ledwith	
Hazel McAuliffe	
Cait McCarthy	

Clinical Teachers – Dental Hygiene

Martina Collins
Ann Holohan
Caroline Horgan
Claire Murphy
Ann O'Keeffe

Dental Hygienist

Caroline McCarthy   Postgraduate Orthodontic Clinic

Dental Nurse Tutors

Mary Harrington   Clinical
Siobhán Murray

Radiographers

Helen Nwokoeye
Margaret O'Brien   Senior

General Support Services

Abraham Brennan   Security
Jenny Noonan   CSSD
Hilary O'Riordan   CSSD
Marie Kiely   CSSD
John O'Sullivan   Store

ORAL HEALTH RESEARCH SERVICES CENTRE STAFF, 2013
Current and/or Core Personnel

Professor Helen Whelton, Director
Emeritus Professor Denis O'Mullane, Consultant
Dr Mairéad Harding, Lecturer and Researcher (seconded from HSE)
Dr Carmel Parnell, Researcher (seconded from HSE)
Dr Patrice James, Researcher
Dr Marie Tuohy, Researcher (seconded from HSE National Oral Health Lead office)
Dr Makiko Nishi, Ph.D student
Eileen MacSweeney, Laboratory Technician
Virginia Kelleher, Research Assistant
Maria Tobin, Projects Manager
Susan O'Donovan, Office Manager
Liz Flynn, Senior Executive Assistant/PA to Director
Kate McSweeney, Marketing and Communications Manager, College of Medicine and Health

Previous and/or Casual Personnel, 2012/13

Dr Helena Guiney, Ph.D Student (now awarded) and Researcher
Dr Deirdre Browne, Ph.D Student (now awarded) and Researcher
Dr Liam Lynch, Ph.D Student (now awarded)
Dr Rose Kingston, Ph.D Student and Clinical Examiner
Dr Caoimhe O'Shea, Clinical Examiner
Dr Mairéad Browne, Clinical Examiner
Dr John Aherne, Clinical Examiner
Theresa O'Mahony, Dental Surgery Assistant and Research Assistant
Jean Conway, Clinical Study Coordinator
Nuala Hegarty, Dental Hygienist and Assistant Clinical Study Coordinator
Helen Callanan, Dental Hygienist and Assistant Clinical Study Coordinator
Nora O'Mahony, Assistant Clinical Study Coordinator
Michelle Seward, Dental Surgery Assistant
Michelle Coleman, Dental Surgery Assistant and Assistant Clinical Study Coordinator
Eimear Ferguson, Receptionist
Colette Cunningham, Qualitative Researcher
Mairéad McLoughlin, undergraduate dental student, HRB Summer Student Scholarship

The National University of Ireland.

UNIVERSITY COLLEGE, CORK.

AUTUMN EXAMINATIONS, 1913.

SECOND DENTAL EXAMINATION.

PHYSIOLOGY.

Professor Barry ; Professor Milroy.

1. Give a classification of the carbohydrates, naming examples of each class commonly used as foodstuffs.
Describe the changes undergone by these foodstuffs during digestion and absorption.

2. Give a detailed description of the microscopic anatomy of a human tooth, with a short reference to the developmental history of its various parts.
Illustrate your answer by diagrams.

3. Describe the cardiac cycle in man.

4. How would you make and stain a film-preparation of the blood ?
Describe the appearances of the various forms of corpuscles which would be seen in such a preparation of normal human blood.

C 179

The National University of Ireland.

UNIVERSITY COLLEGE, CORK.

AUTUMN EXAMINATIONS, 1913.

SECOND DENTAL EXAMINATION.

ANATOMY.

Professor F. G. Parsons ; Professor D. P. FitzGerald.

1. Describe carefully the alveolar process of the superior maxillary bone, referring especially to the shape, depth, and other characters of the teeth-sockets.

2. Describe the course and relations of the lingual branch of the trigeminal nerve.

3. Describe the main course of the blood-vessels that carry blood to and from the tongue.

4. Describe broadly the structure, course, and important relations of the trachea.

5. Name the muscles attached to the humerus, and give their nerve-supply.

6. Give a general account of the intestinal canal from the pylorus to the beginning of the rectum.

C 180

continued over

D 4 **A**

The National University of Ireland.

UNIVERSITY COLLEGE, CORK.

AUTUMN EXAMINATIONS, 1915—PASS.

B.D.S. Degree Examination.

DENTAL SURGERY.

MR. J. HACKETT, M.B., B.CH.; MR. G. W. CONNOR, M.R.C.S.

1. Discuss at least two of the complications that may arise during or after the extraction of the third mandibular molar.

2. What is Polypus of the gum? Minutely describe the condition. How do you distinguish it from Polypus of the Pulp?

3. What are the conditions that cause Necrosis of the jaw? How would you treat an ordinary case of Necrosis?

4. What is a Ranula? Give the differential diagnosis.

5. Describe in detail a method you would employ to bleach a tooth.

6. How does Arsenic devitalize a tooth? What precautions must be taken when using it for this purpose?

C 145

The National University of Ireland.

UNIVERSITY COLLEGE, CORK.

AUTUMN EXAMINATIONS, 1915.

B.D.S. Degree Examination.

MECHANICAL DENTISTRY.

MR. GEORGE SHEEDY, L.D.S.I.;
MR. GEORGE W. CONNOR, M.R.C.S.

1. Describe in detail how you would proceed to make an interdental splint in a case of compound fracture of the mandible.

2. How are dentures retained in the mouth?

3. How would you make a special impression tray?

4. What are the advantages and disadvantages of a combination gold and vulcanite denture?

5. What is the difference between a velum and an obturator, and give the indications for use of either in cleft-palate work?

6. Describe fully the process of vulcanization of rubber.

C 146

OLLSCOIL NA hÉIREANN, CORCAIGH
UNIVERSITY COLLEGE CORK
SUMMER EXAMINATION 2013
ANATOMY
PAPER 2
AN1006

Prof. S. McClure
Dr. D.S. Barry
Prof. J. Cryan

INSTRUCTIONS FOR ANSWERING PAPER 2

- Attempt all 4 essay questions

- Answer each question in the answer books provided

- Write your name and student number on the front of your answer book

WRITE YOUR NAME
HERE:_____
WRITE YOUR STUDENT NUMBER
HERE:_____

Question 1. Give an account of the palate (hard and soft) by describing its bony structure, foramina, muscles and neurovasculature [20 marks]

Question 2. Write short notes on **both** of the following [20 marks]

(a)   The muscles of the orbit [10 marks]
(b)   The stomach [10 marks]

Question 3. Give an account of the muscles of mastication by describing their origins, insertions, actions and neurovasculature [20 marks]

Question 4. Write short notes on **both** of the following [20 marks]

(a)   The axilla of the upper limb [10 marks]
(b)   The temporomandibular joint [10 marks]

OLLSCOIL NA hÉIREANN, CORCAIGH
THE NATIONAL UNIVERSITY OF IRELAND, CORK

COLÁISTE NA hOLLSCOILE, CORCAIGH
UNIVERSITY COLLEGE, CORK

SUMMER EXAMINATION, 2013

INTRODUCTION TO PHYSIOLOGY

PHYSIOLOGY - PL1030

Please note Exam papers NOT to
leave the Exam Hall

EXTERNAL EXAMINER - PROFESSOR B. LUMB
HEAD OF DEPARTMENT – PROFESSOR K. O'HALLORAN
Lecturer(s) – Dr. F. Markos / Dr. P.T. Harrison / Dr. V. Healy / Dr. T. Ruane-O'Hora

DENTAL 1

THREE HOURS

SECTION A   (75 Marks)

Attempt THREE questions.

1.   Describe how cardiac output is regulated in the body.

2.   Describe how breathing is regulated to maintain normal oxygen and carbon dioxide levels in blood.

3.   Discuss the role of hormones and feedback in the regulation of testosterone production and release.

4.   Write an essay on the role of the liver in digestion.

5.   Write an essay on the physiology of Blood Groups.

6.   Write an essay to explain the role of the Na/Glu Symporter in oral rehydration therapy.

SOURCES & INDEX

SOURCES

Chapter 1

PRIMARY SOURCES: Cork Dental Hospital Staff Meeting Minutes (CDHSMM), vol. 1; Gamble; Assorted Cork city directories, 1846–1921; 1901 and 1911 Census Ireland; North Infirmary Annual Report 1912 (Gamble Papers); **INTERVIEWS:** Ronnie Hackett; **SECONDARY PUBLICATIONS:** Borgonovo; Cameron; Chernin; Cohen; Cummins; Dunne; Epstein; Fleetwood (1983); Fleetwood (1990); Geary; Horgan; Jones and Malcolm; Ann Keogh; John B. Lee (1992); J.J. Lee; McCartney; Miskell; Murphy; O'Rahilly; O'Sullivan; Ross; Scher; Smyth and Cottell; Tomes; White and O'Shea.

Chapter 2

PRIMARY SOURCES: Meeting Minutes of the Cork Dental Students' Society; CDHSMM, vol. 1, vol. 2; North Infirmary and Dental Hospital Annual Report 1938 (courtesy Michael Lenihan); Cork Dental Hospital 1945 Prospectus (Gamble Papers); Ray Gamble Interview (UCC Archives); UCC Calendar, 1926–27, 1931–32 (UCC Archives); *Cork Examiner*, 9, 10, 12, 14, 16 Sept., 21 Oct. 1925; *Irish Times*, 9, 16, 21 Oct. 1925, 17 Mar. 1945; *Irish Independent*, 27 Oct. 1930, 21 June 1932; *Irish Press*, 25 Apr. 1932, 17 May 1933; **INTERVIEWS:** Pat Gleeson, Joe Power; **OTHER WRITTEN MATERIAL:** Eddie Scher; **SECONDARY PUBLICATIONS:** Adams; Cohen; Coleman; Dickson; Gamble; Horgan; Jones and Malcolm; Ann Keogh; Dermot Keogh; John B. Lee (1971); McCluggage; Moody and Beckett; Murphy; O'Grada; O'Rahilly; O'Sullivan; Scher; Sherlock; Sognnaes.

Chapter 3

PRIMARY SOURCES: CDHSMM, vol. 2, vol. 3; Brian Barrett, 'The Dental School' (Brian Barrett Papers); *Irish Press*, 7 July 1949; *Irish Independent*, 15 Nov. 1954, 15 Dec. 1960, 19 July 1961; *Irish Times*, 11 Dec. 1948, 9 Apr., 17 Oct. 1949, 27 Jan. 1953, 15 Nov. 1954, 10, 12 Oct. 1956, 12 Oct. 1959, 3 Nov. 1962, 3 Feb., 30 Nov., 1964; **INTERVIEWS:** Brian Barrett, Hugh Barry, Vincent Bluett, Chris Collins, Ger Fitzgerald, Pat Gleeson, Theresa O'Mahoney, Brian O'Riordan, Willie Palmer, Joe Power, Tim Riordan, Eddie Scher; **WRITTEN CONTRIBUTIONS:** Hugh Barry; **OFFICIAL PUBLICATIONS:** 'Teviot Report'; 'Report of the Committee Appointed by the Medical Faculty, University College Cork, To Consider Clinical Teaching in the Cork Hospitals'; 'Report on Visitation', General Dental Council, 1961; 'Summary of Structure of the Staff of the Dental Schools'; **SECONDARY PUBLICATIONS:** Cohen; Cummins; Delaney; Dickson; Dunne; Gamble; John B. Lee (1971); John B. Lee (1992); McCarthy; McCluggage; Moody and Beckett; Murphy; O'Mullane and Whelton; O'Sullivan; Russell; Sherlock; Sognnaes.

Chapter 4

PRIMARY SOURCES: Meeting Minutes of the Munster Branch of the IDA; CDHSMM, vol. 3, vol. 4; *Dáil Éireann Parliamentary Debates*: vol. 239, no. 8, Thurs. 27 Mar. 1969; vol. 246, no. 8, Wed. 13 May 1970; vol. 247, no. 10, Thurs. 18 June 1970; vol. 262, no. 7, Tues. 11 July 1972; vol. 263, no. 7, Thurs. 9 Nov. 1972; vol. 267, no. 6, Thurs. 12 July 1973; vol. 268, no. 5, Thurs. 25 Oct. 1973; vol. 270, no. 11, Thurs. 28 Feb. 1974; vol. 276, no. 10, Thurs. 12 Dec. 1974; vol. 277, no. 12, Tues. 6 Feb. 1975; vol. 278, no. 6, Thurs. 20 Feb. 1975; vol. 296, no. 11, Wed. 16 Feb. 1977; vol. 301, no. 8, Thurs. 17 Nov. 1977; vol. 304, no. 3, Thurs. 28 Feb. 1978;

vol. 328, no. 11, Thurs. 7 May 1981; Barrett Papers: 'Memorandum for UCC President on Proposed New Cork Dental Hospital, 25 January 1966'; Working Party Report on University Reorganisation in so far as it Relates to Dental Teaching, January 1973'; 'The Dental School'; 'New Dental School Correspondence'; 'Cork Hospitals Project Summary, September 1968'; 'Comments on the Booklet "Dental Teaching Hospitals in Ireland" Presented by the Staff Association of the Dublin dental hospital October 1975, by Brian Barrett and Michael Kelleher, 7 Nov. 1975'; Cork University Dental School and Hospital, 'Developments which led to the Assumption of Responsibility for the Control and Management of the Hospital by University College Cork'; Assorted Student Strike flyers; *Cork Examiner*, 9 Apr., 15 May, 1 Oct. 1981, 21 June 1983; *Evening Echo*, 14 May 1981, 6 Mar. 1982, 20 Aug. 1983; *Irish Independent*, 13, 14, 19 May, 18 Nov. 1970, 5 Aug. 1972, 9 Jan., 27 June, 27 Nov. 1973; **INTERVIEWS:** Brian Barrett, Hugh Barry, Chris Collins, Dan Finn, Michael Kelleher, Brian O'Riordan, Tim Riordan, Gordon Russell, Noel Walsh, Tom Walsh; **OFFICIAL PUBLICATIONS:** 'Commission on Higher Education 1960–67 Report'; 'Report on University Reorganisation'; 'Irish Dental Association Meeting Plenary Addresses'; 'A Formal Report on the Need for a Dental School in Cork, Presented to the Minister for Education by the Irish Dental Association with Special Reference to the Higher Education Authority Report'; 'A Memorandum to the Ministers for Education and Health on the State of Dental Education in the Republic of Ireland'; 'Joint Working Party Report'; **SECONDARY PUBLICATIONS:** Barrett and Corkery; Cohen; Dunne; Gamble; Kaim-Caudle; Lee (1972) (1992); McCarthy; Moody and Beckett; Murphy; O'Sullivan; Russell; Sherlock; Smyth and Cottell.

Chapter 5

PRIMARY SOURCES: Meeting Minutes of the Munster Branch of the Irish Dental Association; Barrett Papers: Dental Council Of Ireland Visitation of the First Dental Exams, 1994–1995, Report of the Visitors, CUDSH Academic Plan, 1991–1996; 'New Dental School Correspondence'; *Dáil Éireann Parliamentary Debates*: vol. 365, no. 8, Wed. 23 Apr. 1986; vol. 373, no. 3, Thurs. 4 June 1987; vol. 405, no. 3, 19 Feb. 1991; vol. 409, no. 4, Wed. 5 June 1991; **INTERVIEWS:** Una Atkins, Brian Barrett, Peter Cudmore, Seamus Hickey, Michael Kelleher, Theresa O'Mahoney, Gordon Russell, Noel Walsh; **WRITTEN CONTRIBUTIONS:** Finbarr Allen, Fiona Graham, Joe Hallissey, Mary Harrington, Mary Hegarty, Christine McCreary, Donal McDonnell, Gerry McKenna, Declan Millett, Kathryn Neville, Conor O'Brien, Anne O'Keefe, Eleanor O'Sullivan, Noel Ray, Cillian Twomey, Noel Walsh; **OTHER WRITTEN MATERIAL:** Anne Aiken, Dr. Edith Allen, Claire Barry, Gerry Bradley, John Browne, Richard Browne, Frank Burke, P.J. Byrne, Joe Clarkson, Peter Cooney, Terry Cullinane, Claire Cronin, Frank Daly, Robert Ellwood, Mark Foley, Dario Gio, Michael Hannah, Ailish Hannigan, Clare Horgan, Professor Martin Kinirons, Joe Lemasney, Professor Marion McCarthy, Seán McCarthy, Professor Robbie McConnell, George McSweeney, Bill Murphy, Catherine Nevin, Kathryn Neville, Brian O'Connell, Theresa O'Mahony, Collette O'Sullivan, Eleanor O'Sullivan, Robin O'Sullivan, Professor Duncan Sleeman, Killian Twomey; **SECONDARY PUBLICATIONS:** Gamble; Graham/Kinirons/Holland; Holland/Kenefick/O'Mullane; John B. Lee (1992); Murphy; O'Mullane and Whelton; O'Sullivan.

Chapter 6

PRIMARY SOURCES: BDS Final Year Exam Papers, 1913–2013; Assorted UCC Calendars, 1911–2013; **INTERVIEWS:** Hugh Barry, Ger Fitzgerald, Pat Gleeson, Joe Power, Brian O'Riordan, Tim Riordan; **WRITTEN MATERIAL:** Edith Allen, Professor Finbarr Allen, Sharon Curtin, Professor Martin Kinirons, Professor Marion McCarthy, Gerry McKenna, Eleanor O'Sullivan, Joe Lemasney, Kathryn Neville, Professor Duncan Sleeman; **SECONDARY PUBLICATIONS:** Gamble; Gutmann; John B. Lee (1992); Murphy; Smyth and Cottell.

Chapter 7

PRIMARY SOURCES: Gamble taped interview; *Irish Independent,* 14 Jan. 1954; *Irish Times,* 22 Oct. 1992; **INTERVIEWS:** Una Atkins, Hugh Barry, Chris Collins, Dan Finn, Ger Fitzgerald, Tim Holland, Barry Johnson, Brian O'Riordan, Joe Power, Sarah Kate Quinlivan, Noel Walsh; **WRITTEN MATERIAL:** John Browne, Richard Browne, Claire Cronin, Miriam Crowley, Mark Foley, Pat Harnett, Charlie Haly, Mary Kiely, Mary McCarthy, Bill Murphy, Professor Nuala Porteus, D Vaughan, **OFFICIAL PUBLICATIONS:** 'Cork University Dental School and Hospital 100 Years of Dental Evolution Centenary Conference Programme'; **SECONDARY PUBLICATIONS:** Colbert; Gamble; Murphy.

Epilogue

WRITTEN CONTRIBUTIONS: Professor Finbarr Allen, Professor Martin Kinirons, Professor Nairn Wilson; **WRITTEN MATERIAL:** Seryth Colbert, Kathryn Neville; **OFFICIAL PUBLICATIONS:** 'Cork University Dental School & Hospital Review'.

INDEX: Photographs

Riordan, Tim 76, 83
Roche, Michael 33
Röntgen, Wilhelm Conrad 5
Royal Army Dental Corps (RADC) 30–1
Royal College of Surgeons in Ireland 8, 71, *passim*
    Irish Committee for Specialist Training in
        Dentistry 106
Royal College of Surgeons of England 8, *passim*
Royal Dental Hospital (London) 8
Russell, J. Gordon 56–7, 99, 101, 132
Russell, Seán 85
Ryan, Bríd 149–51, 158

Sanderson, F.M.H. 10
Scher, Edwin 47
Scher, Eric 46–50, 53
    Dr Eric Scher Prize 47
Scher, Gerald 46
Scher, Israel 6–7, 10, 12, 25, 29, 33, 36–7, 45–6,
    49, 100
Scher, Ivor 46–7
Scher, Leslie 46, 48, 50, 53
Sequah (Native American medicine man) 5
Shalloe, Liam 156
Shalloe, Patricia 156
Sheedy, George 10, 12, 25
Sisk, John, and Son building contractors 81
Sisters of Charity of St Vincent de Paul 12, 32–4
    Revd Mother Raphael 32
    Sr Ann 35
    Sr Brendan 32–3, 35
    Sr Josephine 12, 35
    Sr Monica (Mary McCarthy) 34–5
    Sr Vincent 35
    St Theresa 35
Sleeman, Duncan 98, 135
Smiddy, Alf 173, 175
Southern Health Board 77, 80, 102–4, *passim*
Spain, Bernie 103
Spillane, Amelia 142
St Finbarr's Hospital dental clinic 104
Straumann Co. 98
Sullivan, Stanley 10
Sullivan, T.S. 12

Teehan, Charlie 158
Teviot Report (1944) 50
Trinity College Dublin (TCD) 8, 67–9, 71,
    105, 165
Twomey, Cillian 173, 175
Twomey, Eithne 132

Unilever Co. 115
    Unilever Dental Research Group 116
University College Cork (UCC) 2, 9–11, 26,
        61, 67, 69–70, 74–5, 116, *passim. See
        also* Queen's College Cork
    Academic Staff Association 70
    College of Medicine and Health 88–9, 109
    Comhairle Teacthi Na Mac Léinn 96
    Department of Education and Science 122
    Ionad Bairre 122
    Ladies' Club 145
    Men's Club 20, 145
    School of Medicine 26, 69, 73, 82
University College Dublin (UCD) 8, 6–68, 71.
        See also University of Dublin
    School of Medicine and Medical Science 100
University of Birmingham 8–9
University of Dublin 8. *See also* University
        College Dublin (UCD)
University of Limerick Medical School 165

Vaughan, Eugene David 163

Walsh, Noel 69, 85, 94, 96–7
Walsh, Tom 60–1
Ward, Terrence 162
War of Independence 16–18
Warren, Emma 100
Waterford Institute of Technology 111
Whelan, Eugene 13, 128
Whelton, Helen 115–17, 165
White, Zita 111
Wiley, Arthur C. 10, 12
Windle, Sir Bertram 9–11, 18, 26, 120, 175
Wren, John 30–1
Wren, William 30